Pocket Guide to

Commonly Prescribed Drugs

a LANGE medical book

Glenn N. Levine, MD
Section of Cardiology
University Hospital
Boston University Medical Center
Boston, Massachusetts

Pharmacology Editor

Robert L. Barkin, M.B.A., PharmD, N.H.A.
Assistant Director of Pharmacy
Assistant Professor, Rush Medical College
Rush-Presbyterian-St. Luke's Medical Center
Chicago, Illinois

APPLETON & LANGE
Norwalk, Connecticut

Prentice Hall International (UK) Limited, *London*
Prentice Hall of Australia Pty. Limited, *Sydney*
Prentice Hall Canada, Inc., *Toronto*
Prentice Hall Hispanoamericana, S.A., *Mexico*
Prentice Hall of India Private Limited, *New Delhi*
Prentice Hall of Japan, Inc., *Tokyo*
Simon & Schuster Asia Pte. Ltd., *Singapore*
Editora Prentice Hall do Brasil Ltda., *Rio de Janeiro*
Prentice Hall, *Englewood Cliffs, New Jersey*

ISBN: 0-8385-8023-8
ISSN: 1063-7168

Acquisitions Editor: Martin Wonsiewicz
Production Editor: Sheilah Holmes

PRINTED IN THE UNITED STATES OF AMERICA

Dedicated to the overworked, underappreciated
interns, residents, and medical students
of the health care system

Table of Contents

Preface

The *Pocket Guide to Commonly Prescribed Drugs* is a comprehensive, easy-to-use reference to the essential information needed for prescribing medications safely and effectively. Drugs are listed alphabetically, with all information for each drug contained within its individual listing. There is no need to search through a table of contents or index, to turn from chapter to chapter, to consult confusing charts, or to seek cross-referenced information.

In recognition that medical practitioners are hard pressed for time, each listing has been kept as concise as possible with only the most clinically relevant information included. Comprehensive, easy-to-understand information is included for each drug, presented under clearly labeled subheadings for quick retrieval. This includes the following:

- Initial, loading, and maintenance doses
- Commercially available preparations
- Mechanisms of action and therapeutic uses
- How the drug is cleared from the body, whether dose adjustments are necessary in patients with hepatic or renal failure, and whether supplemental doses are necessary after hemodialysis or peritoneal dialysis
- Important side effects
- Relative and absolute contraindications to use
- Relative and absolute cost
- Clinically useful "pearls," including information to tell the patient about the drug, suggested physical and laboratory evaluation before beginning therapy, the drug's potency or efficacy compared with therapeutically similar drugs, blood levels to monitor during therapy, the drug's effects on laboratory tests, which drugs need to be tapered when discontinuing therapy, pregnancy category, and many other useful bits of information

Besides comprehensive prescribing information, The *Pocket Guide to Commonly Prescribed Drugs* places special emphasis on providing information to help prevent iatrogenic complications when using each medication. This information includes

- Whether or not, and how the dosage or dosing interval should be adjusted in patients with liver or kidney disease
- Important interactions the drug may have with other drugs
- Contraindications to use, and under what circumstances the drug must be used with caution
- Risk of using the drug during pregnancy

Listings have been reviewed by specialists in cardiology, endocrinology, gastroenterology, general internal medicine, hematology, infectious diseases, intensive care medicine, nephrology, neurology, oncology, psychiatry, pulmonary medicine, and rheumatology. The entire content has been reviewed by professor of pharmacology Dr. Robert Barkin.

The *Pocket Guide to Commonly Prescribed Drugs* should prove useful to a wide variety of health care providers, including interns and residents, medical students, primary care physicians, nurses and nurse practitioners, physician assistants, podiatrists, dentists, and other health related professionals.

I hope that this book will help you, the medical practitioner, to prescribe drugs with confidence and safety, and thus to optimize your patients' medical care.

G.N.L.

Please send comments and suggestions to:

Dr. Glenn N. Levine
Section of Cardiology
University Hospital
Boston University Medical Center
88 East Newton Street
Boston, MA 02118

Acknowledgments

I am thankful and indebted to many individuals for their editing, suggestions, assistance, and support.

For review of drugs in their various specialties to Elaine Alpert, Dino Beer, Elizabeth Buonoane, Dave Cave, James Gilbert, Warren Hershman, Paul Heusketh, Benton Idelson, Carlos Kase, Rafael Kieval, Mike Klein, Tom Lamont, Stu Levitz, Ron McCaffrey, Cindy McCrone, James Melby, Phil Podrid, Burt Polansky, Joseph Radazzo, David Salant, Bill Stenson, Joe Torre, Sumar Varma, Evar Vosberg, and Don Weiner.

For suggestions and support to Dave Faxon, Kathi Henry, Tom Lamont, Norman Levinsky, Carol O'Malley, and John Wilson.

For editing, comments, suggestions, and advice to Robert Barkin.

For manuscript editing to Nancy Megley.

For supervising publication of the *Guide* to Anne-Marie Zwierzyna.

And for continuous and enthusiastic support and guidance, and for serving as outstanding professional and personal role models, to Gary Balady, Dave Battinelli, Warren Hershman, and Burton Polansky.

Introduction

This book is designed to be a pocket reference to medications commonly used in clinical medicine. It is not intended to be all inclusive, but rather to list some of the common and clinically important pharmacologic properties of each drug. Information contained in the *Guide* was compiled from a variety of sources. There is some variation in the literature and among specialists on certain aspects of the clinical profile for many drugs. Listed in this book are what the author considers to be reasonably well accepted and agreed upon information for each agent.

Drugs are generally listed by their generic name, in capital letters, and are cross-referenced by trade name; combination drugs are generally listed by trade name. Information included for most drugs consists of dosing schedules, mode of clearance, dosage adjustments necessary in renal failure, liver disease, and following dialysis, side effects, drug interactions, contraindications, relative cost, therapeutic blood levels, serum values that should be monitored during therapy, pregnancy category, and other clinically useful "pearls." The information provided in each section, and how to use it, is as follows.

The **Dose** section lists, where relevant, the initial, loading, and maintenance or usual dose of each drug. For some drugs, the dosing schedule often depends on the route of administration or the specific disease being treated. Doses given are those for adult patients; dosing schedules for children usually differ and are given only for those drugs commonly prescribed for children.

The **Preparations** section lists available forms, sizes, and concentrations of each medication.

The **Actions** section lists the pharmacologic or physiologic action of the drug, and what it is used for. Additional information on the mechanism of action is provided where appropriate.

The **Clearance** section describes major modes of elimination for the drug, usually by various degrees of liver metabolism and renal excretion. The section gives general guidelines on dosing changes in renal dysfunction, as listed in the chart below, and whether dosage adjustments are necessary in patients with liver disease. The section also lists whether enough drug is removed by hemodialysis (HD) or peritoneal dialysis (PD) to require supplemental doses after dialysis.

Designation	**GFR = 10–50 ml/min**	**GFR < 10 ml/min (ESRD)**
"no change"	No adjustment necessary	No adjustment necessary
"slight"	Give 75–100% the usual dose or increase the dosing interval up to 1½ times the normal interval	Up to 2 times the normal interval
"moderate"	Give 50–75% the usual dose or increase the dosing interval to ≈½–2 times the normal interval	Give only 25–50% the usual dose or increase the dosing interval to ≈2–4 times the normal interval
"marked"	Give ≤50% the usual dose or increase the dosing interval to ≈2–4 times the normal interval	Give <25% the usual dose or increase the dosing interval to 2–4 times the normal interval

The **Side Effects** section lists some of the more common or more clinically important side effects associated with each drug. This section is *not* designed to list every reported side effect of each medication; reported side effects that occurred with similar frequency in control groups, and thus did not appear to be causally related to the medication, are usually not included.

The **Drug Interactions** section lists important interactions that the listed drug has with other medications. Interactions include reciprocal effects on serum level of the listed drug or drugs taken with it; increased metabolism of the listed drug through induction of hepatic enzymes by other drugs; and effects of the listed drug on prothrombin time (PT) in patients taking warfarin.

The **Cautions** section lists some of the clinically important contraindications and relative contraindications to the use of each drug.

The **Pearls** section lists clinically useful information for the drug, beginning with its relative cost (as explained in the next paragraph). Also included in the "Pearls" section are, where appropriate, blood levels to monitor, cautions with use, onset and duration of action, and therapeutic levels. At the end of this section the FDA-designated pregnancy category (explained below), when available, is given.

The relative cost of each drug is denoted as one to four dollar signs ($), with each drug somewhat arbitrarily rated into one of the four categories that best describes its cost. Wholesale prices are listed for many intravenous and inpatient drugs. The amount billed to the patient (or insurance provider) varies widely from hospital to hospital, and depends largely on purchasing agreements between the hospital and pharmaceutical companies; the markup may be several times the wholesale price. Average retail costs are based on a survey of August 1991 prices in representative retail-chain pharmacies in the New England area. Prices for both generic and brand-name drugs are provided. Cost rating criteria are as follows:

$: Inexpensive
Affordable to patients on even a limited income; inexpensive when compared to other drugs with similar functions.

$$: Should be affordable to most patients
Cost should generally not be a significant concern when using or prescribing this drug.

$$$: Somewhat or relatively expensive
May be difficult for many patients to afford (if not adequately covered by insurance); cost may be a consideration when using or prescribing this drug; consider using less expensive drugs with similar actions or functions.

$$$$: Expensive in both relative and absolute terms
Cost should be considered when using or prescribing this drug; consider using (substantially) less expensive drugs with similar actions or functions.

Brief summaries of each pregnancy category are listed below. For medications which do not have an FDA-established pregnancy category, important information may nevertheless be available to guide prescribing decisions, and *PDR* or other sources should be consulted.

Category A: Controlled studies in women have failed to demonstrate a risk to the first-trimester fetus, and the possibility of fetal harm appears remote.

Category B: (1) Animal studies have not shown a fetal risk but there are no controlled studies in pregnant women, *or* (2) animal studies have shown an adverse effect that was not confirmed in controlled studies of women.

Category C: (1) Studies in animals have revealed adverse effects on the fetus but there are no controlled studies in women, *or* (2) studies in women and animals are not available. Drugs in this category should be given only if the potential benefit justifies the potential risk to the fetus.

Category D: There is positive evidence of human fetal risk, but the benefits from use in pregnant women may be acceptable despite the risk.

Category X: Studies in animals, humans, or both have demonstrated fetal abnormalities, and the risk of using the drug in pregnant women clearly outweighs any possible benefit. The drug is contraindicated in women who are pregnant or potentially pregnant.

Pocket Guide to Commonly Prescribed Drugs

Abbokinase Open-Cath: *see* **UROKINASE**

Accupril: *see* **QUINAPRIL**

Accutane: *see* **ISOTRETINOIN**

ACEBUTOLOL (Sectral)

Dose: Initial, 200 mg PO bid; may increase to 600–1200 mg PO daily in divided doses. Maximum daily dose in elderly patients, 800 mg.

Preparations: 200 and 400 mg capsules.

Actions: β_1-Selective β-blocker; used to control PVCs.

Clearance: Excreted via GI tract; active metabolite diacetolol is excreted mainly by the kidney.
Markedly reduce dosage in impaired renal function.
Use with caution in liver disease.

Side Effects: Fatigue, dizziness, dyspnea, bradycardia, hypotension, heart failure.

Cautions: Contraindicated in severe bradycardia, overt cardiac failure or cardiogenic shock, and second- or third-degree AV block.
Use with caution in reactive airway disease.

Pearls: When discontinuing, taper gradually to avoid "β-blocker withdrawal."
Pregnancy category B.

ACETAMINOPHEN (Tylenol; *see also* Darvocet, Fioricet, Percocet, Tylenol with Codeine, Vicodin, Vicodin ES)

Dose: Preparation dependent.

Regular-strength: One or two 325 mg tablets PO q4–6h; max, 12 tablets in 24 h.

Extra-strength: Two 500 mg tablets PO q6–8h; max, 8 tablets in 24 h.

Rectal: 650–1000 mg q4–6h prn; max, 4,000 mg daily.

Liquid: 30 mL (2 Tbsp) of Extra-Strength Tylenol liquid q4–6h prn; max, 4000 mg (4 doses) in 24 h.

Preparations: 325 and 500 mg tablets; 325 and 650 mg suppositories; 8 oz bottles of Extra-Strength Tylenol liquid containing 500 mg/15 mL (1 Tbsp).

Actions: Analgesic and antipyretic; used to treat pain and fever.

Clearance: Metabolized via liver.

Slightly increase dosing interval in impaired renal function (metabolites can accumulate).

Avoid in significant liver disease.

Supplemental dose suggested after HD but not after PD.

Side Effects: Hepatotoxicity at overdose level and with chronic use of 4–8 g daily.

Cautions: Avoid in liver disease.

Pearls: Cost $ (100 tablets retail: generic ≈$3, Tylenol ≈$6).

Hepatotoxicity is rare if >10 g ingested (unless patient has history of alcohol abuse); fatalities rare if >15 g ingested.

Early symptoms of overdose include nausea and vomiting, diaphoresis, anorexia, and general malaise.

Clinical and laboratory evidence of hepatotoxicity may not become apparent until 48–72 h after ingestion.

Marked "synergistic" liver toxicity with alcohol.

ACETAZOLAMIDE (Diamox)

Dose: Disease dependent.

Congestive heart failure: 250–375 mg PO or IV qd; raising dosage does not increase diuresis.

Metabolic alkalosis: 500 mg PO or IV q8h.
Glaucoma: 500 mg (SR capsule) PO bid.

Preparations: 125 and 250 mg tablets; 500 mg sustained-release capsules.

Actions: Carbonic anhydrase inhibitor with mild diuretic properties; used to treat CHF, metabolic alkalosis, and glaucoma. In the kidney, causes loss of HCO_3^- ion (which carries off Na^+, K^+, and H_2O), resulting in alkalization of the urine.

Clearance: Primarily renal excreted.
Slightly increase dosing interval in impaired renal function; avoid in ESRD.
Clearance is reduced in elderly patients.

Side Effects: Paresthesias (especially tingling), hearing dysfunction, changes in appetite, GI disturbances, fever, rash, anaphylaxis, bone marrow depression, hemolytic anemia, decreased WBCs and platelets, Stevens-Johnson syndrome.

Cautions: Contraindicated in patients with cirrhosis (increases risk of hepatic encephalopathy), decreased serum levels of Na^+ or K^+, marked liver or kidney dysfunction, hyperchloremic acidosis, or adrenal insufficiency. Patients allergic to sulfonamides can have cross-sensitivity allergic reactions to acetazolamide.
Contraindicated in pregnant or potentially pregnant patients.

Pearls: Cost \$–\$\$ (100 tablets retail: generic ≈\$8, Diamox ≈\$37).
Use with caution in COPD (can aggravate acidosis).
Periodically check CBC.
Alternate-day therapy may increase response by allowing the kidney to recover.
Contraindicated during pregnancy.

ACETYLCYSTEINE (N-ACETYLCYSTEINE, Mucomyst)

As mucolytic or as therapy for acetaminophen overdose

Mucolytic

Dose: 3–5 mL of 20% solution in nebulizer (or 6–10 mL of 10% solution) tid–qid or prn.

Actions: Mucolytic that decreases viscosity by theoretically "opening" disulfide linkages; actual clinical role, if any, is highly controversial.

Side Effects: Bronchospasm, stomatitis, nausea, rhinorrhea.

Pearls: Cost $$ ($\approx$$6 wholesale per treatment).
  Pregnancy category B.

Acetaminophen Overdose

Dose: 140 mg/kg loading dose PO or via NG tube, then 17 doses of 70 mg/kg PO or via NG tube q4h.

Actions: Prevents liver injury in acetaminophen overdose (most likely by restoring glutathione levels).

Side Effects: Rare urticaria. The nitrogen load in N-acetylcysteine can exacerbate hepatic encephalopathy and necessitate dosage reduction.

Pearls: Cost $$ ($\approx$$40 wholesale for loading dose and 17 treatments).
  Do not give concurrently with activated charcoal (which absorbs it).
  Repeat any dose that is vomited within 1 h of administration.
  May be administered by duodenal intubation if necessary.
  In suspected overdose do *not* wait for serum level determinations before starting therapy.
  Pregnancy category B.

ACETYLSALICYLIC ACID (ASPIRIN, ASA, ENTERIC COATED ASPIRIN, Ecotrin, ZORprin)

Dose: Disease dependent.
  Cardiovascular disease: 325–1000 mg qod–qd.
  Rheumatologic disease: Up to 1 g PO qid.

Preparations: 325 and 500 mg tablets; Ecotrin is enteric coated aspirin; ZORprin is controlled-release aspirin.

Actions: Antipyretic, anti-inflammatory, analgesic, antiplatelet, and antithrombotic agent that irreversibly inhibits platelet aggregation; used to treat fever, pain, cardiovascular disease, and cerebrovascular disease.

Clearance: Metabolized via liver; renal excreted.

Avoid in ESRD.

Modify dosing regimen when used for chronic therapy in liver disease.

Supplemental dose suggested after HD or PD.

Side Effects: GI irritation, nausea and vomiting, tinnitus, metabolic acidosis, respiratory alkalosis, ARDS, occult GI bleeding.

Cautions: Use with caution, if at all, in patients with liver dysfunction, impaired renal function, elevated uric acid, history of salicylate sensitivity or asthma, or nasal polyps.

Use with caution in patients taking warfarin.

Avoid in children or teenagers with varicella or other viral infections.

Pearls: Cost $ (100 tablets retail: generic ≈$2, brands ≈$5, generic coated ≈$5, Ecotrin ≈$7).

Regular use is frequently associated with heme (+) stools without a significant lesion in the GI tract; overt ulceration without symptoms can also occur.

Signs and symptoms of overdose (salicylism) include tinnitus, vertigo, headache, confusion, drowsiness, sweating, hyperventilation, diarrhea, and vomiting.

Pregnancy category D.

Actifed (PSEUDOEPHEDRINE + TRIPROLIDINE)

Dose: 1 tablet or capsule PO q4–6h; max, 4 tablets or capsules in 24 h.

Actions: Combination decongestant and antihistamine; used to treat nasal congestion and rhinorrhea.

Side Effects: Drowsiness, excitability (especially in children).

Cautions: May be contraindicated in patients taking MAOI.

Use with caution in hypertension, diabetes, heart disease, thyroid disease, glaucoma, or benign prostatic hypertrophy.

Pearls: Cost $ (pack of 24 tablets ≈$4 wholesale).

Caution patients to avoid driving or ingesting alcohol while taking this product.

Antihistamines are useful only in allergic rhinitis and serve no therapeutic function with infection-mediated symptoms.

Actifed Plus (PSEUDOEPHEDRINE, TRIPROLIDINE + ACETAMINOPHEN)

Dose: 2 caplets or tablets PO q6h; max, 8 caplets or tablets in 24 h.

Actions: Combination decongestant, antihistamine, and analgesic/antipyretic; used to treat upper respiratory tract infections.

Side Effects: Drowsiness, excitability (especially in children).

Cautions: May be contraindicated in patients taking MAOI. Use with caution in patients with hypertension, diabetes, heart disease, thyroid disease, glaucoma, benign prostatic hypertrophy, or significant liver damage.

Pearls: Cost $ (pack of 20 tablets ≈$3 wholesale).

Caution patients to avoid driving or ingesting alcohol while taking this product.

Antihistamines are useful only in allergic rhinitis and serve no therapeutic function with infection-mediated symptoms.

Activase: see TISSUE PLASMINOGEN ACTIVATOR

ACTIVATED CHARCOAL: see CHARCOAL

Acutrim: see PHENYLPROPANOLAMINE

ACYCLOVIR (Zovirax)

Dose: Disease dependent.

Mucocutaneous lesion: 5% ointment q3h 6 times daily.

Genital herpes: 200 mg PO q4h 5 times daily without regard to meals.

Herpes zoster (shingles): 800 mg PO q4h 5 times daily without regard to meals.

Severe genital herpes: 5 mg/kg IV q8h.

Herpes simplex encephalitis: 5–10 mg/kg IV q8h.

Shingles in immunocompromised host: 10 mg/kg IV q8h.

Preparations: 200 and 800 mg capsules; 500 mg vials for injection; 3 and 15 g containers of 5% ointment.

Actions: Antiviral agent that inhibits DNA synthesis; used to treat HSV-I, HSV-II, varicella zoster, and EB virus infection.

Clearance: Predominantly renal excreted.

Moderately increase dosing interval in impaired renal function; give 200 mg PO q12h or 2.5 mg/kg/d IV in ESRD.

No change in dosage needed for liver disease.

Supplemental dose suggested after HD.

Side Effects: Route dependent. PO: Nausea and vomiting. IV: Local phlebitis, rash, transient rise in serum creatinine, rare CNS changes (1%).

Pearls: Cost $$$$ (PO ≈$5–9/d retail for 200 mg tablets, ≈$25/d retail for 800 mg tablets!; IV ≈$120/d wholesale).

Patients should be well hydrated to avoid renal tubule crystallization.

Pregnancy category C.

ADENOSINE

Dose: Initial, 6 mg IV; if no response, may give 12 mg IV.

Preparations: 6 mg/2 mL vials for injection.

Actions: Antiarrhythmic; used to treat SVT. Acts as (−) dromotropic (reduces conduction) but not (−) inotropic.

Clearance: $t_{1/2}$ is 30 sec; extensively degraded in the body.

Side Effects: Facial flushing, transient chest pain or pressure, dyspnea, decreased HR, reflex tachycardia, reinitiation of SVT, dizziness, anaphylactoid reactions.

Drug Interactions: Dipyridamole decreases its uptake and markedly delays its clearance. Methylxanthines, theophylline, and caffeine all block adenosine receptors and reduce its effectiveness.

Pearls: Cost $$ (≈$12–30; IV verapamil is much less expensive).

Usually will terminate SVT but not VT.

Works within 30 sec.

Inject *quickly,* preferably through a large-bore or central IV catheter.

Pregnancy category C.

ADH: *see* VASOPRESSIN

Adriamycin: *see* DOXORUBICIN

Adsorbocarpine: *see* PILOCARPINE

Advil: *see* IBUPROFEN

Afrin: *see* OXYMETAZOLINE

ALBUMIN

Dose: 25 g IV initially, then as indicated by clinical situation.

Preparations: Available in 5% and 25% solutions.

Actions: Albumin preparation that increases plasma osmotic pressure; used to treat peripheral or pulmonary edema, in certain cases of shock, and by some physicians during paracentesis.

Side Effects: Febrile reactions, nausea and vomiting, increased salivation.

Cautions: Contraindicated in severe anemia or CHF.

ALBUTEROL (Proventil, Ventolin)

Dose: Route dependent.
   Nebulizer: 0.25–0.5 mL of 0.5% solution in 3 mL NS.
   Metered-dose inhaler: 2 inhalations q4–6h (the Rotohaler inhaler contains no fluorocarbons).
   Regular-acting PO: 2–4 mg tid–qid; max, 8 mg daily.
   Long-acting PO: 4–8 mg of long-acting tablets (Proventil Repetabs) q12h.

Preparations: 2 and 4 mg regular tablets; 4 mg long-acting tablets; 17 g inhaler canisters.

Actions: β_2-Selective stimulant; used to treat reactive airway disease.

Side Effects: Tachycardia, palpitations, tremor, cough and bronchospasm, nausea, hypokalemia, restlessness, anxiety.

Drug Interactions: MAOI and tricyclics increase its vascular effects (use with caution). Antagonized by β-blockers.

Cautions: Use with caution in patients with CAD, hypertension, or tachyarrhythmias.

Pearls: Cost $$$ (Provental inhaler ≈$23 retail each, 2 mg tablets $6–$25 wholesale/100 tablets).
   Pregnancy category C.

Aldactazide (HYDROCHLOROTHIAZIDE + SPIRONOLACTONE)

Dose: 25–200 mg PO daily of each component, given qd or in divided doses.

Preparations: Available in two pill sizes, one containing 25 mg each and the other 50 mg each of spironolactone and hydrochlorothiazide.

Actions: Combination diuretic with K^+-sparing properties; used to treat hypertension.

Pearls: Cost $$$$ (≈$2/d retail).
   Pregnancy category not established.

Aldactone: see SPIRONOLACTONE

Aldomet: see METHYLDOPA

Alkeran: see MELPHALAN

Allerest (CHLORPHENIRAMINE + PHENYLPROPANOLAMINE)

Dose: Regular tablets: 2 PO q4h prn; max, 8 tablets in 24 h; SR caplets: 1 PO q12h prn.

Actions: Combination antihistamine and sympathomimetic; used to treat upper respiratory tract infections.

ALLOPURINOL (Zyloprim)

Dose: Initial, 100 mg PO qd; may increase by 100 mg at weekly intervals until serum uric acid reaches <6 mg/dL. Usual, 200–300 mg PO qd.

Preparations: 100 and 300 mg tablets.

Actions: Xanthine oxidase inhibitor that decreases uric acid production; used to treat gout.

Clearance: Allopurinol and its oxidized metabolite oxypurinol are renal excreted.

Moderately to markedly reduce dosage or increase dosing interval in impaired renal function.

No change in dosage needed for liver disease.

Side Effects: Precipitation of acute gout attack, drowsiness, nausea and vomiting, elevated LFTs, skin rash (discontinue immediately to avoid progression to Stevens-Johnson syndrome and toxic epidermal necrosis).

Drug Interactions: Dramatically reduce dosage of mercaptopurine or azathioprine (Imuran) when given concurrently. Decreases renal excretion of chlorpropamide.

Pearls: Cost $ (generic ≈$4.50/mo retail, Zyloprim ≈$12/mo retail).

Give colchicine when allopurinol is started (to decrease likelihood of precipitating gout attacks).

Discontinue immediately if the following symptoms appear (signifying severe systemic reaction): fever, chills, nausea and vomiting, skin rash, itching, painful urination, hematuria, eye irritation, or swelling of lips or mouth.

Pregnancy category C.

ALPHA INTERFERON: see INTERFERON

ALPRAZOLAM (Xanax)

Dose: Initial, 0.25–0.50 mg PO tid; max, 4–6 mg PO daily.

Preparations: 0.25, 0.5, 1.0, and 2.0 mg tablets.

Actions: Benzodiazepine analog; used to treat anxiety and panic attacks.

Clearance: Metabolized via liver; renal excreted.

No change in dosage needed in impaired renal function; use with caution in ESRD (can cause sedation and encephalopathy).

Side Effects: Drowsiness.

Drug Interactions: Raises serum levels of tricyclics. Potentiates CNS depressant effects of other CNS depressants. Cimetidine, isoniazid, propoxyphene, propranolol, metoprolol, and ketoconazole increase its effectiveness.

Pearls: Cost $$ (0.5 mg ≈$60 retail/100 tablets).

Withdrawal seizures can occur with abrupt discontinuance after even relatively brief use.

Prolonged use is associated with physical dependence.

Pregnancy category D.

Altace: see RAMIPRIL

ALTEPLASE: see TISSUE PLASMINOGEN ACTIVATOR

ALternaGEL: see ALUMINUM HYDROXIDE

ALUMINUM CARBONATE (Basaljel)

Dose: 15–30 mL, 2 tsp, or 2–4 tablets or capsules with or after meals and qhs; max, 24 capsules, 24 tablets, or 24 tsp in 24 h.

Preparations: Standard-dose capsules; standard-dose scored tablets; 12 oz suspension.

Actions: Antacid that reduces intestinal absorption of phosphorus; usually used to treat hyperphosphatemia in ESRD.

Side Effects: Constipation.

Drug Interactions: Reduces effectiveness of tetracyclines.

Pearls: Cost $ ($10 wholesale/100 tablets).

Pregnancy category C.

ALUMINUM HYDROXIDE (ALternaGEL or Amphojel; see also Maalox, Mylanta)

ALternaGEL

Dose: 1–2 tsp prn between meals and qhs.

Preparations: 5 and 12 oz bottles.

Actions: Antacid that lacks laxative properties of magnesium-containing antacids.

Side Effects: Constipation.

Pearls: Cost $$ (12 oz bottle ≈$7.50 retail).

Amphojel

Dose: 30–60 mL, two 300 mg tablets, or one 600 mg tablet PO tid with meals.

Preparations: 300 and 600 mg tablets; 12 oz bottles of 320 mg/5 mL (1 tsp) unflavored and peppermint-flavored suspension.

Actions: Antacid that reduces intestinal absorption of phosphorus; usually used to treat hyperphosphatemia in ESRD.

Side Effects: Constipation.

Pearls: Cost $$ (12 oz bottle ≈$6 retail; tablets ≈$0.30/d retail).

ALUMINUM PHOSPHATE (Phosphaljel)

Dose: 15–30 mL PO q2h between meals and qhs.

Side Effects: Constipation.

Drug Interactions: Reduces effectiveness of tetracyclines.

Pearls: Cost $$ (12 oz bottle ≈$6 retail).
  Pregnancy category C.

Alupent: *see* METAPROTERENOL

AMANTADINE (Symmetrel)

Dose: Disease dependent.

Parkinsonian and extrapyramidal symptoms: 100 mg PO bid initially; may raise slowly to 300–400 mg daily given in divided doses.

Influenza A virus infection: 200 mg PO qd; if CNS side effects develop, may give 100 mg PO bid instead.

Preparations: 100 mg capsules and tablets; 16 oz bottles containing 50 mg/5 mL (1 tsp) syrup.

Actions: (1) Antiparkinsonian agent that increases neuronal release of dopamine and other catecholamines and delays presynaptic reuptake of these neurotransmitters; used to treat parkinsonism. (2) Antiviral agent; used in prevention and treatment of influenza A.

Clearance: Renal excreted.

Markedly increase dosing interval and reduce dosage in impaired renal function.

No change in dosage needed for liver disease.

Supplemental dose not required after HD.

Significantly decrease dosage in elderly patients.

Side Effects: Dose-related dizziness, light-headedness, blurred vision, anxiety, irritability, hallucinations, confusion, depression, ataxia, increased seizure activity, headache, anorexia, constipation, CHF, orthostatic hypotension, elevated LFTs, dry mouth, peripheral edema, reversible livedo reticularis.

Drug Interactions: Potentiates CNS depressant effects of other CNS depressants. Produces increased atropine-like effects when used with anticholinergic agents.

Pearls: Cost $$$ (100 tablets ≈$86 retail).

Onset of action within 48 h.

Discontinue gradually to prevent withdrawal reactions.

Use with caution in patients with history of seizures or liver disease

Signs and symptoms of overdose include urine retention, hyperactivity, convulsions, arrhythmias, hypotension, acid-base disturbances, and acute toxic psychosis.

Sometimes used to treat fatigue in patients with multiple sclerosis.

Pregnancy category C.

AMIKACIN

Dose: Loading, 7.5 mg/kg IV; maintenance, 5 mg/kg q8h or 7.5–10 mg/kg q12h IM or IV.

Preparations: 100 and 500 mg vials for injection.

Actions: Bactericidal aminoglycoside antibiotic that irreversibly inhibits protein synthesis. Excellent aerobic gram (−) coverage including *Pseudomonas;* not effective against anaerobes.

Clearance: Renal excreted.

Markedly decrease dosage or increase dosing interval in impaired renal function.

No change in dosage needed for liver disease.

Supplemental dose suggested after HD or PD.

Side Effects: Nephrotoxicity, ototoxicity, rare increased neuromuscular blockade.

Drug Interactions: Concomitant use with cephalothin, vancomycin, cisplatin, amphotericin B, nitrogen mustard compounds, loop diuretics, and cyclosporin all increase risk of nephrotoxicity or ototoxicity. Can inactivate mezlocillin, azlocillin, and pipercillin if given concurrently.

Pearls: Cost $$$$ ($2000/wk wholesale); consider using significantly less expensive gentamicin.

Used primarily in patients with gentamicin- and tobramycin-resistant organisms.

(+) CSF penetration in meningeal inflammation.

Follow peak and trough levels.

Pregnancy category D.

AMILORIDE (Midamor; *see also* Moduretic)

Dose: 5–10 mg PO qd–bid.

Preparations: 5 mg tablets.

Actions: K$^+$-sparing diuretic; used to treat hypertension.

Clearance: Metabolized via liver; renal excreted.
Avoid if CrCl <50 mL/min.
May need to adjust dosage in liver disease.

Pearls: Cost $ (≈$0.30/d retail).

AMINOPHYLLINE

Dose: Loading, 5–6 mg/kg (ideal weight) IV over 30 min; maintenance, 0.5–0.6 mg/kg/h (ideal weight).

Preparations: 250 and 500 mg vials for injection.

Actions: Respiratory agent with bronchodilating, diaphragmatic stimulating, and probably other actions; used to treat reactive airway disease.

Clearance: Metabolized via liver.
No change in dosage needed in impaired renal function.
Significantly increase dosing interval or significantly reduce dose in liver dysfunction; significantly reduce dosage in liver disease.
Supplemental dose suggested after HD or PD.

Side Effects: Markedly increased HR, palpitations, arrhythmias, headache, seizures, coma, nervousness, irritability, nausea and vomiting, diarrhea, reflux (because of decreased lower esophageal sphincter tone), tachypnea, rash.

Drug Interactions: Antagonistic to propranolol. Cimetidine, fluoroquinolones, and erythromycin raise its serum level. Ketoconazole, dilantin, and isoproterenol decrease its serum level.

Pearls: Cost $.
IV dose (in mg/h) can be calculated by dividing total daily PO dose by 20 (e.g., 300 mg PO bid = 600 mg PO daily; 600 divided by 20 yields an IV dose of 30 mg/h).
Therapeutic range is usually defined as 10–20 μg/mL.
Risk of toxicity is increased when serum level >20 μg/mL.
$t_{1/2}$ is decreased in smokers and in patients taking phenytoin. $t_{1/2}$ is increased in the elderly and in patients with CHF, COPD, liver disease, viral infection, or high fever.
Pregnancy category C.

AMIODARONE (Cordarone)

Dose: Disease dependent.

Ventricular arrhythmias: 800–1,600 mg PO daily for 1–3 weeks, then 400–800 mg PO daily for 1–3 weeks, then 200–400 mg daily (some physicians will use higher maintenance doses).

Atrial fibrillation (not FDA approved for this at present): 600 mg PO daily for 1 week, then 400 mg daily for 2 weeks (consider trial of electrical cardioversion at this point); maintenance dose if converts, 200 mg PO qD.

Preparations: 200 mg tablets.

Actions: Type III antiarrhythmic; used to treat VT and SVT.

Clearance: Metabolized via liver; metabolites are active; significant enterohepatic recirculation and hepatobiliary excretion occur.

No change in dosage needed in impaired renal function.

There are no studies examining the need to reduce dosage in liver dysfunction.

Supplemental dose not required after HD.

Side Effects: Arrhythmias, CHF, significantly reduced HR, conduction abnormalities, headache, malaise, fatigue, tremor, neuropathy, GI (nausea and vomiting, constipation, anorexia, elevated LFTs, hepatitis), pulmonary fibrosis, corneal microdeposits, hypothyroidism or hyperthyroidism, elevated thyroid function tests, photodermatitis.

Drug Interactions: Raises serum levels of digoxin and antiarrhythmics. Can potentiate β-blocker and calcium antagonist mediated bradycardia, sinus arrest, or AV block. Prolongs PT in patients taking warfarin.

Cautions: Use with caution with β-blockers and general anesthetics (can cause decreased BP and HR, conduction abnormalities, and CHF).

Pearls: Cost $$$$ (≈$260 retail/100 tablets).

Obtain chest x-ray and liver and thyroid function tests every 6 months.

Pregnancy category C.

AMITRIPTYLINE (Elavil)

Dose: (for depression)

Initial, 75 mg PO daily in divided doses or 50–100 mg PO qhs; maintenance, 40–150 mg PO qhs.

Preparations: 10, 25, 50, 75, 100, and 150 mg tablets.

Actions: Tricyclic antidepressant with sedative effects; used to treat depression and other disorders, including painful neuropathies and chronic fatigue syndrome.

Clearance: Metabolized via liver.
No change in dosage needed in impaired renal function.
Substantially reduce dosage in elderly patients.
Supplemental dose not required after HD or PD.

Side Effects: Atropine-like effects, sedation, cardiovascular effects, decreased WBCs, elevated or decreased glucose, hypersensitivity reactions, conduction abnormalities.

Drug Interactions: Hyperpyrexia when used with MAOI, anticholinergic agents, or neuroleptics. Paralytic ileus when used with anticholinergic agents. Cimetidine raises its serum level.

Cautions: Contraindicated in patients who have taken MAOI within 2 weeks.
Use with caution in elderly patients and in patients with history of seizures, cardiovascular disease, hyperthyroidism, urine retention, angle-closure glaucoma, or increased intraocular pressure.

Pearls: Cost: generic $, Elavil $$ (100 tablets retail: 50 mg generic ≈$10, 50 mg Elavil ≈$65).
Signs and symptoms of overdose include confusion, seizure, coma, visual hallucinations, dilated pupils and ocular dysmotility, hypothermia or hyperpyrexia, arrhythmias, decreased conduction and bundle-branch block, CHF, hypotension, muscle rigidity, and hyperreflexia.
Pregnancy category not established.

AMOXAPINE (Asendin)

Dose: Initial, 50 mg PO tid or 150 mg PO qhs; may gradually increase to maximum of 400–600 mg daily in patients without history of seizures. Usual, 200–300 mg daily.

Preparations: 25, 50, 100, and 150 mg tablets.

Actions: Antidepressant; used to treat depression.

Clearance: Metabolized via liver to a dopamine receptor antagonist neuroleptic.

No change in dosage needed in impaired renal function.

Reduce dosage in elderly patients.

Side Effects: Sedation, postural hypotension, anticholinergic effects.

In theory, tardive dyskinesia and neuroleptic malignant syndrome can develop.

Cautions: Contraindicated in patients taking MAOI. Use with caution in patients with history of seizures.

Pearls: Cost $$$$ (100 tablets retail: 50 mg ≈$100, 150 mg ≈$300).

Taper dose when discontinuing.

Signs and symptoms of overdose are predominantly neurologic, including seizures.

A small percentage of patients may develop renal failure, particularly ATN secondary to myoglobinuria, 2–5 days after an overdose.

Pregnancy category C

AMOXICILLIN (Amoxil; *see also* Augmentin)

Dose: 250–500 mg PO tid without regard to meals.

For uncomplicated cystitis, may give high-dose therapy (3 g PO qd for 1–3 days).

Pediatric dose: For otitis, sinusitis, pharyngitis, or GU infection, children weighing 8–20 kg, 20 mg/kg daily in 3 divided doses given q8h; children ≥20 kg (44 lb), 250 mg PO q8h. For lower respiratory tract infection, children weighing 8–20 kg, 40 mg/kg daily in 3 divided doses given q8h; children ≥20 kg (44 lb), 500 mg PO q8h.

Preparations: 250 and 500 mg capsules; 125 and 250 mg chewable tablets; 5, 80, 100, and 150 mL bottles containing 125 mg/5 mL (1 tsp) suspension; 5, 80, 100, and 150 mL bottles containing 250 mg/5 mL (1 tsp) suspension.

Actions: Bactericidal penicillin antibiotic that inhibits cell wall synthesis. Some gram (+) coverage including strep and most enterococci (but *not* most staph); some gram (−) coverage including *E. coli, Salmonella,* most *H. influenzae,* some *Proteus,* and some *Klebsiella* but *not Shigella* or β-lactamase–producing organisms (including some *H. influenzae*); some anaerobic coverage.

Clearance: Primarily renal excreted.

Slightly to moderately increase dosing interval in impaired renal function.

No change in dosage needed for liver disease.

Supplemental dose suggested after HD but not after PD.

Side Effects: GI discomfort, diarrhea, abdominal cramps, rash, anaphylactic reaction, allergic interstitial nephritis.

Cautions: Contraindicated in patients with penicillin allergy.

Pearls: Cost $ (≈$8/wk retail).

Tolerated better than oral ampicillin.

Use ampicillin (or other appropriate antibiotics) to cover *Shigella.*

With the emergence of resistant *H. influenzae,* most sources no longer consider amoxicillin adequate therapy for sinusitus and instead recommend Augmentin, Bactrim, or Ceclor.

Pregnancy category B.

Amoxil: see AMOXICILLIN

Amphojel: see ALUMINUM HYDROXIDE

AMPHOTERICIN B

Dose: Disease dependent.

Systemic illness: Give 1 mg IV test dose (with premedication) over 30 min, then 0.20–0.25 mg/kg on the first day; may increase by 0.1–0.2 mg/kg daily to a maximum of 0.5–1.0 mg/kg/d.

Bladder irrigation: Sources vary; regimens include: (1) 15–50 mg in 1 L sterile water as continuous irrigation over 24 h; (2) 50 mg daily in 1 L sterile water as continuous irrigation for 3–5 days; (3) 5–15 mg in sterile water q6–8h for 3–5 days.

Preparations: Injection preparation containing 50 mg powder per vial.

Actions: Polyene antibiotic that alters membrane permeability; used to treat fungal infections.

Clearance: Metabolic pathways unclear but presumed hepatic metabolism; 2–5% excreted unchanged in urine.

Slightly increase dosing interval in ESRD; no change needed in milder renal dysfunction.

May need to reduce dosage in liver disease.

Supplemental dose not required after HD or PD.

Side Effects: Nephrotoxicity, electrolyte wasting (especially K^+ and Mg^{++}), fever and shaking chills (usually 15 min after injection), nausea and vomiting, anorexia, malaise, generalized body pain, myalgias, arthralgias, dyspepsia, diarrhea, local phlebitis, normocytic normochromic anemia, bronchospasm, lymphocytosis, thrombocytopenia, CHF.

Drug Interactions: Corticosteroids can exacerbate K^+ wasting. Other nephrotoxic agents and nitrogen mustard can increase its nephrotoxicity.

Pearls: Cost $ (≈$40 wholesale for 2 weeks of IV therapy).

In critically ill patients, some sources recommend proceeding directly to maximum dose after initial test dose.

Give slowly IV over 4–6 h.

Carefully follow K^+, Mg^{++}, renal function, CBC, and LFTs.

Premedicate with Tylenol or ASA, diphenhydramine 25–50 mg PO or IV, and hydrocortisone 25–50 mg IV (to reduce side effects). Over time, may be able to give without premedication.

Nephrotoxicity may be reduced by prehydration, salt loading, and keeping the patient well hydrated.

Meperidine 50 mg is useful if chills develop.

Pregnancy category B.

AMPICILLIN (see also Unasyn)

Dose: Route dependent.

PO: 250–1000 mg qid 30 min before or 2 h after meals.

IM or IV: 0.5–2 g q6h.

May give high-dose therapy (3.5 g PO qd for 1–3 days) for uncomplicated cystitis.

Oral absorption can be affected by food.

Preparations: 250 and 500 mg tablets; suspensions at various concentrations; powder for injection.

Actions: Bactericidal penicillin antibiotic that inhibits cell wall synthesis. Some gram (+) coverage including strep and entero-cocci (but *not* most staph); some gram (−) coverage including *E. coli*, most *H. influenzae*, *Shigella*, and *Salmonella* (but *not* β-lactamase–producing bacteria, including some *H. influenzae*); some anaerobic coverage. Also effective against *Listeria*, an important cause of meningitis in elderly patients, which cephalosporins do not cover.

Clearance: Some liver metabolism; primarily renal excreted.
Slightly to moderately increase dosing interval in impaired renal function.
No change in dosage needed for liver disease.
Supplemental dose suggested after HD but not after PD.

Side Effects: GI discomfort, rash, anaphylactic reaction, allergic interstitial nephritis.

Cautions: Contraindicated in patients with penicillin allergy.

Pearls: Cost $ (PO ≈$7/wk retail, IV ≈$70/wk wholesale).
Is often preferred for oral use (because of its tid dosing schedule and because its absorption is not affected by food).
Pregnancy category B.

AMRINONE (Inocor)

Dose: Initial, 0.75 mg/kg bolus over 2–3 min; may be repeated 30 min later. Maintenance, 5–10 μg/kg/min.
Doses up to 40 μg/kg/min may be used for refractory CHF.

Preparations: 5 mg/mL injection.

Actions: Positive inotropic agent with vasodilator effects; used to treat CHF.
Hemodynamic effects include increases in cardiac index and BP, decreases in pulmonary vascular resistance, pulmonary capillary wedge pressure, and HR.

Clearance: Metabolized via liver; renal excreted.

Slightly decrease dosage in ESRD; no change needed in milder renal impairment.

Reduce dosage in liver disease.

Side Effects: Increased PVCs and ischemia, hypotension, allergic reactions, mild reduction in platelets (secondary to reduced $t_{1/2}$ of platelets), nausea and vomiting, abdominal pain, rare hepatotoxicity.

Drug Interactions: Can produce hypotension when used with disopyramide.

Pearls: Cost $$$$ ($\approx$$600/d wholesale).

Inotropic effects are additive with digoxin.

Pregnancy category C.

Anafranil: see CLOMIPRAMINE

Ancef: see CEFAZOLIN

ANISTREPLASE (APSAC, Eminase)

Dose: 30 unit IV bolus over 2–5 min.

Preparations: 30 unit vials.

Actions: Thrombolytic; used to treat acute MI. Enzyme is activated after deacylation of the protective anisoyl group, leading to both clot-specific and non-clot-specific conversion of plasminogen to plasmin with resulting thrombolysis.

Side Effects: Bleeding, arrhythmias, hypotension (10%), intracranial bleeding (0.57%), anaphylactic reaction (0.2%).

Cautions: Contraindicated in patients with active internal bleeding, history of CVA, recent intracranial or intraspinal surgery or trauma, severe uncontrolled hypertension, known bleeding diathesis, and intracranial AVM, aneurysm, or neoplasm.

Relatively contraindicated in patients with history of cerebrovascular disease, recent GI or GU bleeding, recent trauma, markedly elevated BP, acute pericarditis, SBE, hemorrhagic retinopathy, age >75 years, septic thrombophlebitis, occluded and infected arteriovenous cannula; patients taking warfarin; or patients with a high likelihood of left heart thrombus.

Pearls: Cost $$$$ ($1700).

Consider giving ASA simultaneously and heparinizing 4–6 h after the anistreplase bolus.

Pregnancy category C.

Antabuse: see DISULFIRAM

Antivert: see MECLIZINE

Anusol suppositories and ointment

Dose: Route dependent.

Rectal suppository: 1 bid and after each evacuation.

Ointment: Apply and rub into cleansed and dried anal tissue q3–4h.

Preparations: 1 and 2 oz tubes; boxes of 12, 24, and 48 suppositories.

Actions: Suppositories contain bismuth, benzyl benzoate, peruvian balsam, and zinc oxide; they relieve pain, itching, and discomfort from hemorrhoids.

Ointment contains benzyl benzoate, peruvian balsam, zinc oxide, and the local analgesic pramoxine hydrochloride; it relieves pain, itching, and discomfort from hemorrhoids.

Anusol-HC: see HYDROCORTISONE SUPPOSITORIES

Apresoline: see HYDRALAZINE

APSAC: see ANISTREPLASE

ARA-C: see CYTOSINE ARABINOSIDE

Aristocort A: see TRIAMCINOLONE ACETONIDE cream, lotion, and ointment

Artane: see TRIHEXYPHENIDYL

ASA: see ACETYLSALICYLIC ACID

Asendin: *see* **AMOXAPINE**

ASPIRIN: *see* **ACETYLSALICYLIC ACID**

ASTEMIZOLE (Hismanal)

Dose: 10 mg PO qd, taken on an empty stomach.

Preparations: 10 mg scored tablets.

Actions: Long-acting antihistamine that blocks H_1 receptors; used to treat allergic conditions.

Clearance: Metabolized via liver; excreted primarily in feces.

Side Effects: Minimal increase in drowsiness (compared with control patients), fatigue, initial increase in appetite and weight gain, dry mouth.

Pearls: Cost $$$ ($\approx$$1.50/d retail), similar to daily cost of Seldane.
Should be taken on an empty stomach to increase bioavailability.
Pregnancy category C.

Atarax: *see* HYDROXYZINE

ATENOLOL (Tenormin)

Dose: Route dependent.
PO: 50–200 mg qd.
IV in acute MI: 5 mg over 5 min; repeat dose 10 min later.

Preparations: 25, 50, and 100 mg tablets; 5 mg/10 mL ampules for injection.

Actions: β_1-Selective β-blocker; used to treat angina and hypertension.

Clearance: Renal excreted; no liver metabolism.
Moderately reduce dosage in impaired renal function.
No change in dosage needed for liver disease.
Supplemental dose suggested after HD but not PD.

Side Effects: Cardiovascular (CHF, markedly decreased HR, AV block, postural hypotension), CNS (vertigo, fatigue, depression, lethargy), bronchospasm, impotence.

Cautions: Relatively contraindicated in patients with greater than first-degree AV block, CHF, or reactive airway disease.

Pearls: Cost $$$ (PO ≈$1.00/d retail).

May cause fewer CNS effects than other β-blockers (because of its low lipid solubility).

Taper when discontinuing (abrupt discontinuance can cause rebound reactions).

Pregnancy category C.

ATROPINE (see also Lomotil)

Dose: 0.5–1.0 mg IV; may repeat as indicated to maximum of 2.0 mg.

Preparations: Various concentrations for injection.

Actions: Antimuscarinic; used primarily to treat symptomatic bradycardia. Also used in therapy for insecticide poisoning.

ATROPINE eye drops (Isopto Atropine)

Dose: Instill 1 or 2 drops (written "gtt") in the eye up to qid for iritis.

Preparations: 0.5, 1.0, and 3.0% solution; 0.5 and 1.0% ointment.

Actions: Cycloplegic; used to treat iritis.

Side Effects (systemic): Dry mouth, tachycardia, fever, delirium.

Pearls: To decrease systemic absorption, compress the lacrimal sac with a finger after instilling drops.

Atrovent: see IPRATROPIUM

Augmentin (AMOXICILLIN + CLAVULANATE)

Dose: 250–500 mg PO q8h without regard to meals.

Pediatric dose (for otitis media, sinusitis, lower respiratory tract infection): Children weighing <40 kg, 40 mg/kg daily (of amoxicillin component) given in 3 divided doses q8h; for children ≥40 kg, give usual adult dosage.

Preparations: Quantity of amoxicillin (A) and clavulanate (C) components: '250' tablets containing 250 mg A and 125 mg C; '500' tablets containing 500 mg A and 125 mg C; '125' chewable tablets containing 125 mg A and 31.25 mg C; '250' chewable tablets containing 250 mg A and 62.5 mg C; 75 and 150 mL bottles of banana-flavored suspension containing 125 mg A and 31.25 mg C per 5 mL (1 tsp); 75 and 150 mL bottles of orange-flavored suspension containing 250 mg A and 62.5 mg C per 5 mL (1 tsp).

Actions: Semisynthetic bactericidal penicillin antibiotic that inhibits cell wall synthesis, combined with clavulanate, a β-lactamase inhibitor. Good gram (+) coverage including enterococci, strep, and most staph (*not* MRSA); good gram (−) coverage and good anaerobic coverage including *B. fragilis.*

Clearance: Some renal excretion of amoxicillin and clavulanate. Moderately increase dosing interval in impaired renal function. Supplemental dose suggested after HD.

Side Effects: Diarrhea, nausea and vomiting, rash, elevated LFTs, vaginitis.

Cautions: Contraindicated in patients with penicillin allergy.

Pearls: Cost $$$ (≈$50 retail/7–10 days of therapy); *see* Penicillin for a comparison of weekly costs for brand-name and generic oral antibiotics.

Can produce false (+) result on dipstick test for urine glucose.

Increases risk of rash in patients with mononucleosis or taking allupurinol.

Pregnancy category B.

Aventyl: see NORTRIPTYLINE

Axid: see **NIZATIDINE**

Axsain: see **CAPSAICIN cream**

AZATHIOPRINE (Imuran)

Dose: Disease dependent.
Renal transplant patients: Usually 3–5 mg/kg PO or IV qd initially; maintenance, 1–3 mg/kg daily.
Rheumatoid arthritis: Often 1.0 mg/kg PO or IV qd initially, given in 1 or 2 divided doses; may gradually increase to maximum of 2.5 mg/kg daily.

Preparations: 50 mg tablets; 100 mg/20 mL injection.

Actions: Immunosuppressive antimetabolite; used in patients who have received homograft transplants and to treat autoimmune diseases.

Clearance: Cleaved *in vivo* to mercaptopurine. Both it and mercaptopurine are metabolized in the liver and in RBCs; there is little renal excretion.
Slightly decrease dosage in impaired renal function.
One source suggests avoiding azathioprine in liver disease.
Supplemental dose suggested after HD.

Side Effects: Severe leukopenia (dose limiting), macrocytic anemia, decreased platelets, nausea and vomiting, elevated LFTs, hepatitis with biliary stasis, cholestatic hepatotoxicity, pancreatitis, mucositis, restrictive lung disease.

Drug Interactions: Allopurinol markedly reduces its metabolism (substantially decrease the dosage).

Cautions: Contraindicated in pregnant or potentially pregnant patients.

Pearls: Cost $$$$ (PO ≈$2.50/d wholesale).
Should be taken on an empty stomach to enhance absorption.
Usually takes 6–8 weeks for response in rheumatoid arthritis; patients not responding within 12 weeks are considered treatment failures.
Pregnancy category X.

AZITHROMYCIN (Zithromax)

Dose: Disease dependent. Should be taken at least 1 h before or 2 h after meals.

COPD exacerbation, pneumonia, pharyngitis, uncomplicated skin infection: Single dose of 500 mg PO on day 1, then 250 mg PO qd for days 2–5.

Nongonococcal urethritis or cervicitis from *Chlamydia:* Single dose of 1000 mg PO.

Preparations: 250 mg capsules.

Actions: Macrolide antibiotic that inhibits protein synthesis. Has been shown to have in vitro activity against the following organisms, although the clinical significance of this activity for some listed organisms is not established: gram (+) coverage including *S. aureus, S. pyogenes, and Viridans* group strep (but *not* MRSA or enterococci); gram (−) coverage including *H. influenzae* and *H. ducreyi, M. catarrhalis (Branhamella catarrhalis), Campylobacter jejuni,* and *Legionella pneumophila* (but *not* E. coli, *Klebsiella,* or *Proteus);* anaerobic coverage including *Bacteroides bivius, C. perfringens,* and *Peptostreptococci;* other coverage includes *Mycoplasma pneumoniae, Treponema pallidum,* and *Ureaplasma urealyticum.*

Clearance: Metabolized and excreted primarily via liver.

Little data is available on its use in liver or kidney disease, so use with caution in these patients.

Side Effects: Diarrhea, nausea, abdominal pain.

Drug Interactions: Little data is currently available.

Other macrolide antibiotics have been shown to raise serum levels of theophylline, digoxin, carbamazepine, phenytoin, and cyclosporine, to decrease clearance of triazolam (Halcion), and to prolong PT in patients taking warfarin. These effects should be borne in mind when using azithromycin.

Cautions: Contraindicated in patients with history of allergic reaction to any macrolide antibiotic.

Pearls: Cost $$$.

Should not be used for treatment of infections in patients <16 years old.

Pregnancy category C.

Azlin: *see* AZLOCILLIN

AZLOCILLIN (Azlin)

Dose: 3 g IV q4h or 4 g IV q6h.

Preparations: 2, 3, and 4 mg vials for injection.

Actions: Bactericidal antipseudomonal penicillin that inhibits cell wall synthesis. Some gram (+) coverage including strep and enterococci (but *not* staph); excellent gram (+) coverage including *P. aeruginosa;* good anaerobic coverage including *B. fragilis.*

Clearance: Primarily renal excreted.
Slightly increase dosing interval in impaired renal function.
No change in dosage needed for liver disease.
Supplemental dose suggested after HD but not after PD.

Side Effects: Rash, drug fever, hypersensitivity reactions, interstitial nephritis, GI distress, elevated LFTs.

Drug Interactions: Concomitant use with aminoglycosides increases risk of nephrotoxicity.

Cautions: Contraindicated in patients with penicillin allergy.

Pearls: Cost $$$ ($\approx$$85/d wholesale).
Pregnancy category B.

Azmacort: *see* TRIAMCINOLONE

AZT: *see* ZIDOVUDINE

AZTREONAM

Dose: 500 mg–2 g IV q8h; usual, 1 g IV q8h. May give IM up to 1 g q8h.

Preparations: 500 mg, 1 g, and 2 g vials for injection.

Actions: Monobactam bactericidal antibiotic that inhibits cell wall synthesis. Excellent aerobic gram (−) coverage (variable, hospital-dependent *P. aeruginosa* coverage); not active against gram (+) organisms or anaerobes.

Clearance: Primarily renal excreted.
Moderately decrease dosage in impaired renal function.
No change in dosage needed for liver disease.
Supplemental dose suggested after HD.

Side Effects: Eosinophilia (8%).

Cautions: May be contraindicated with other β-lactam antibiotics (actions can be antagonistic).

Pearls: Cost $$$ (≈$40/d wholesale); consider using less expensive gentamicin.
Pregnancy category B.

Azulfidine: see SULFASALAZINE

Bacid: see LACTOBACILLUS

Baciguent: see BACITRACIN

BACITRACIN (Baciguent, Bacitrin; *see also Cortisporin*)

Dose: Apply thin film to skin bid–qid.

Preparations: 0.5 and 1 oz tubes.

Actions: Topical antibiotic that inhibits cell wall synthesis. Good gram (+) coverage; poor gram (−) coverage.

Side Effects: Skin rashes, itching, burning, tingling.

Pearls: Cost $ (1 oz generic ≈$3–4 retail).
Pregnancy category C.

BACLOFEN (Lioresal)

Dose: 40–80 mg daily in divided doses.

Preparations: 10 and 20 mg tablets.

Actions: Muscle relaxant; used to treat spasticity.

Side Effects: Drowsiness, dizziness, weakness, fatigue, confusion, headache, insomnia, urinary frequency, hypotension.

Pearls: Cost $$$ (100 tablets retail: 20 mg generic ≈$55, 20 mg Lioresal ≈$85).

Abrupt withdrawal may cause seizures and hallucinations.

Bactrim, Septra (TRIMETHOPRIM + SULFAMETHOXAZOLE)

Dose: Disease dependent.

Outpatient bronchitis: 1 double-strength (DS) tablet PO bid for 14 days.

Outpatient urinary tract infection: 1 DS tablet PO bid for 7–14 days.

Inpatient urinary tract infection: 5 mg/kg/d trimeth. (with fixed ratio of sulfa. component) IV in 2 or 3 divided doses.

Inpatient non-urinary-tract infection: 8–10 mg/kg/d trimeth. (with fixed ratio of sulfa. component) IV in 3 divided doses.

PCP: 20 mg/kg/d trimeth. (with fixed ratio of sulfa. component) IV in 4 divided doses.

Preparations: Regular and double strength. Each regular-strength tablet contains 80 mg trimethoprim and 400 mg sulfa-methoxazole.

Actions: Antibiotic that blocks the folic acid synthesis pathway. Good gram (+) coverage including strep and staph (but *not* enterococci); good gram (−) coverage including ampicillin-resistant *H. influenzae* (but *not P. aeruginosa*).

Clearance: Some systemic metabolism; renal excreted.

Decrease dosage in impaired renal function.

Reduce dosage in severe liver disease; no change needed for milder liver dysfunction.

Supplemental dose suggested after HD.

Side Effects: Nausea and vomiting, anorexia, cholestasis and hepatitis, pancreatitis, pancytopenia, common allergic reactions, hallucinations, depression, seizure.

Drug Interactions: Can inhibit phenytoin metabolism.

Cautions: Contraindicated in sulfa allergy or G6PD deficiency.

Pearls: Cost $ (PO generic ≈$5/wk retail, PO Bactrim ≈$15–$20/wk retail, IV ≈$10/d wholesale); see under Penicillin for a comparison of weekly costs for brand-name and generic oral antibiotics.

G6PD-deficient patients can develop hemolysis.

May cause *falsely* elevated creatinine measurements.

Check CBC frequently.

PO dose (in mg) is equivalent to IV dose (in mg).

Pregnancy category C.

Basaljel: see ALUMINUM CARBONATE

BECLOMETHASONE nasal inhaler and spray (Beconase, Beconase AQ, Vancenase, Vancenase AQ)

Dose: Delivery dependent.

Beconase and Vancenase: 1 inhalation in each nostril bid–qid.

Beconase AQ and Vancenase AQ: 1 or 2 inhalations in each nostril bid.

Preparations: Beconase and Vancenase: 16.8 g canister containing 200 metered doses. Beconase AQ and Vancenase AQ: 25 g bottle with fitted metering atomizing pump and nasal adaptor.

Actions: Topical steroid; used to treat allergic rhinitis.

Side Effects: Local irritation and burning, sneezing attacks, rare *Candida* infections, systemic absorption, and steroid-mediated side effects.

Pearls: Cost $$$ (inhaler ≈$33–38 retail).

Pregnancy category C.

BECLOMETHASONE oral inhaler (Beclovent, Vanceril)

Dose: 2–4 inhalations PO qid.

Preparations: 16.8 g canister containing 200 metered doses.

Actions: Inhaled steroid; used to treat reversible airway disease.

Side Effects: Oral candidiasis, suppression of adrenal axis, osteoporosis (after chronic high-dose therapy).

Pearls: Cost $$$ (inhaler ≈$30 retail).
Rinsing the mouth after use may decrease side effects.
Pregnancy category C.

Beclovent: see BECLOMETHASONE oral inhaler

Beconase, Beconase AQ: see BECLOMETHASONE nasal inhaler and spray

Benadryl: see DIPHENHYDRAMINE

BENAZEPRIL (Lotensin)

Dose: Initial, 10 mg PO qd (5 mg PO qd if patient is currently taking a diuretic); after 2 weeks may increase to 20 mg PO qd. Max, 20 mg PO bid.

Preparations: 10 and 20 mg tablets.

Actions: Newly developed ACE inhibitor; used to treat hypertension in patients >55 years old (approved for use only in this group at present).

Clearance: Predominantly renal clearance in healthy patients; liver metabolism appears to compensate in patients with renal insufficiency.
No change in dosage needed in mild to moderate renal impairment; for GFR <30 mL/min, begin with 5 mg PO bid.
No change in dosage needed for liver disease.

Side Effects: Hypotension, weakness or fatigue, occasional dizziness. Theoretical decrease in WBCs or cough (based on side effects of other ACE inhibitors).

Cautions: Contraindicated during second and third trimesters of pregnancy.

Pearls: Cost $$–$$$ (5 or 10 mg ≈$67 retail/100 tablets).
Manufacturer claims price is 10–47% less than other ACE inhibitors.

Diuretics potentiate its antihypertensive effects.

Patients taking diuretics and elderly patients are especially prone to first-dose hypotension.

Consider starting therapy at night so that, if BP falls, patients will not be at work or another inconvenient location and can easily lie down.

Pregnancy category D.

Benzac: see BENZOYL PEROXIDE

Benzagel: see BENZOYL PEROXIDE

Benzamycin (BENZOYL PEROXIDE + ERYTHROMYCIN)

Dose: Apply to cleansed, dried skin bid.

Preparations: 23.3 g gel containing 3% erythromycin and 5% benzoyl peroxide.

Actions: Combination antibacterial; used to treat acne vulgaris.

Side Effects: Dry skin, pruritus, allergic reactions, erythema.

Pearls: Cost $$$ (tube ≈$24 retail).

Avoid contact with mucous membranes or inflamed, denuded skin.

Pregnancy category C.

BENZONATATE (Tessalon)

Dose: Usual, 1 "perle" PO tid; max, 6 "perles" in 24 h.

Pill should be swallowed, *not* chewed or allowed to dissolve in the mouth.

Preparations: 100 mg "perles."

Actions: Non-narcotic antitussive that inhibits the cough stimulus by anesthetizing stretch receptors in the lungs and pleura; used to treat persistent cough.

Side Effects: Sedation, dizziness, headache, nasal congestion, skin eruptions and pruritus, GI upset.

Pearls: Cost $$$ (≈$1 retail per "perle").
Pregnancy category C.

BENZOYL PEROXIDE (Benzac, Benzagel, Clearasil, Oxy-5, Oxy-10; *see also* Benzamycin)

Dose: Apply to skin 1–3 times daily.

Preparations: Benzac: 5% and 10% gel preparations containing 12% alcohol in 60 and 90 g containers; Benzagel: 5% and 10% gel preparations containing 14% alcohol in 1.5 and 3 oz containers; Clearasil: 10% lotion in 1 oz squeeze bottle; Oxy-5 and Oxy-10: 5% and 10% lotions in 1 oz plastic bottle.

Actions: Topical antibacterial; used to treat acne vulgaris.

Pearls: Bleaches hair and clothing.
Patients allergic to benzoic acid derivatives may show cross-sensitivity.

BENZTROPINE (Cogentin)

Dose: Disease dependent.
Idiopathic parkinsonism (adjunctive therapy): Initial, 0.5–1.0 mg PO or IM qhs; usual, 1–2 mg PO tid.
Drug-induced extrapyramidal disorder: 1–2 mg PO or IM daily, given qd–tid.

Preparations: 0.5, 1.0, and 2.0 mg tablets; 1 mg/mL injection.

Actions: Synthetic competitive anticholinergic agent that also has antihistaminic and atropine-like effects; used to treat Parkinson's disease and other extrapyramidal disorders.

Clearance: Metabolized primarily via liver.

Side Effects: Numerous CNS effects, tachycardia, constipation, dry mouth, nausea and vomiting, blurred vision, dilated pupils, urine retention, allergic reactions, rash, anhidrosis, hyperthermia.

Drug Interactions: Can cause paralytic ileus or exacerbate psychotic behavior in patients taking phenothiazines or tricyclics. Potentiates CNS depressant effects of other CNS depressants. Antacids and antidiarrheal agents increase its intestinal absorption.

Cautions: Use with caution in patients with arrhythmias, prostate hypertrophy, or wide-angle glaucoma.

Pearls: Cost: generic $$, Cogentin $$1/2 (100 tablets retail: generic ≈$10, Cogentin ≈$25).
Is equally effective IM or IV; may give IV if IM is contraindicated.
Is more effective in treating tremor and rigidity than for bradykinesia.
Pregnancy category not established.

BEPRIDIL (Vascor)

Dose: 200–400 mg PO qd. Allow 10 days between dosage changes.

Actions: Calcium-channel blocker that also blocks the fast sodium channel; used to treat refractory angina.

Clearance: Completely metabolized in the liver; negligible amount excreted unchanged in urine.

Side Effects: Headache, dizziness, nausea and vomiting, negative inotropy, dose-related QT prolongation.

Drug Interactions: Raises serum level of digoxin.

Cautions: Contraindicated in patients with history of ventricular arrhythmias, sick sinus syndrome, second- or third-degree heart block, or cardiogenic shock.

Pearls: Cost $$$.
May be prudent to follow corrected QT interval.
Pregnancy category C.

Betagan: see LEVOBUNOLOL

BETAMETHASONE cream and lotion (many brands;
see also Lotrisone topical cream)

Dose: Apply to skin qd–tid.

Preparations: 15 and 45 g tubes of 0.05–0.1% preparations.

Actions: Potent topical corticosteroid; used to treat many dermatologic conditions.

Pearls: Cost: generic $, Diprolene $$$ (45 g tube: generic ≈$10 retail, Diprolene ≈$45 retail).

Extensive use over prolonged periods, especially with occlusive dressings, may lead to systemic absorption and related side effects of systemic steroids.

BETAXOLOL eye drops (Betoptic)

Dose: Apply 1 drop (written "gtt") bid.

Preparations: 0.5% solution.

Actions: Topical cardioselective β-blocker that decreases production of aqueous humor; used to treat glaucoma.

Side Effects (systemic): Bradycardia, worsening AV block, worsening CHF, bronchoconstriction.

Cautions: Relative or clear contraindications include CHF, sinus bradycardia, second- or third-degree heart block, or history of bronchospastic airway disease.

BETHANECHOL (Urecholine)

Dose: Route dependent.

PO: Initial, 5–10 mg/h until satisfactory response or maximum dose of 50 mg is reached; maintenance, give minimum effective dose (as determined by cumulative initial dose) tid–qid; usual, 10–50 mg tid–qid.

SQ: Initial, 0.5 mL (2.5 mg); repeat every 15–30 min until satisfactory response or maximum of 2.0 mL (10 mg) is reached; maintenance, give minimum effective dose (as determined by cumulative initial dose) tid–qid; usual, 1 mL (5 mg) tid–qid.

Preparations: 5, 10, 25, and 50 mg tablets; 5 mg/mL injection.

Actions: Parasympathomimetic (cholinergic) agent that increases detrusor muscle contraction and stimulates micturition; used to treat nonobstructive urine retention.

Side Effects: Malaise, increased gastric motility and tone, abdominal discomfort, headache, hypotension and reflex tachycardia, flushing, bronchial constriction, lacrimation, miosis, salivation, diarrhea, urinary urgency.

Pearls: Cost: generic $$, Urecholine $$$$ (25 mg generic ≈$0.30/d retail, 25 mg Urecholine ≈$2.70/d retail).

Tablets should be taken 1–2 h after meals to avoid GI distress.

Warn patients about possible orthostatic hypotension-like effects.

Pregnancy category C.

Betoptic eye drops: see BETAXOLOL

Biaxin: see CLARITHROMYCIN

BICARBONATE (SODIUM BICARBONATE)

Dose: Route dependent.

PO: 300–600 mg bid–tid.

IV drip: Mix 2 ampules (88 meq) in 1 liter 0.45% NS (approximately equal to 0.9% solution) at IV rate appropriate for clinical setting.

IV bolus: 1 meq/kg; may give additional 0.5 mg/kg q10–12min as indicated.

Pearls: Use with caution in patients with CHF (carries significant Na$^+$ load).

BISACODYL (Dulcolax)

Dose: Route dependent.

PO: 5–10 mg taken on an empty stomach with water.

PR: 10 mg.

Enema: 37.5 mL.

Preparations: 5 mg enteric coated tablets; 10 mg suppositories; liquid enema preparations.

Actions: Nondiarrheogenic cathartic that stimulates smooth muscle contractions; used to treat constipation.

Pearls: Onset of action 6–10 h PO, 15–60 min PR, immediate when given as enema.

BLEOMYCIN (Blenoxane)

Dose: Tumor dependent. Usually first give a "test dose" in lymphoma patients. One regimen for many malignancies is 0.25–0.50 units/kg (10–20 units/m^2) IV, IM, or SQ weekly or twice weekly.

Preparations: 15 unit vials.

Actions: Antineoplastic agent that inhibits DNA synthesis, and possibly RNA and protein synthesis; used to treat many malignancies.

Clearance: 60–70% renal excreted.
Slightly to moderately reduce dosage in impaired renal function: for patients with serum creatinine of 2.5–4.0 mg/dL, give 1/4 the normal dose; 4.0–6.0 mg/dL, 1/5 the normal dose; 6.0–10.0 mg/dL, 5–10% of the normal dose.
No change in dosage needed for liver disease.
Supplemental dose not required after HD.

Side Effects: Pneumonitis (10%) and pulmonary fibrosis, skin toxicity (erythema, rash, hyperpigmentation, vesiculations, tenderness, etc., usually occurring 2–3 weeks after therapy), rare renal or hepatic toxicity, severe idiosyncratic reaction in 1% of lymphoma patients (hypotension, mental status changes, fever and chills, wheezing).

Pearls: Cost $$$ (15 units $227 wholesale).
Pulmonary fibrosis is the most severe toxicity usually associated with therapy; earliest symptoms and signs are dyspnea and fine rales.
Obtain chest x-rays every 1–2 weeks to look for nonspecific bilateral patchy opacities, usually in lower lung fields.
Decreased total lung volume and vital capacity are the most common abnormalities on pulmonary function tests but do not predict development of pulmonary fibrosis.

DLCO (diffusing capacity) may be a sensitive measure of subclinical pulmonary toxicity; *PDR* recommends checking it monthly.

Pulmonary toxicity increases when cumulative dose exceeds 400 units.

Pregnancy category not established.

Blenoxane: see BLEOMYCIN

Blocadren: see TIMOLOL

Brethaire: see TERBUTALINE inhaler

BRETYLIUM (Bretylol)

Dose: Initial, 5 mg/kg IV; may increase to 10 mg/kg IV over 8 min. Maintenance, 1–2 mg/min IV.

Preparations: 50 mg/mL injection.

Actions: Type III antiarrhythmic; used to treat ventricular tachyarrhythmias.

Clearance: Renal excreted.

Moderately to markedly reduce dosage in impaired renal function; avoid in ESRD.

Dosage change probably unnecessary in liver disease.

Side Effects: Orthostatic hypotension, markedly reduced HR, increased PVCs, nausea and vomiting, diarrhea, vertigo, syncope, confusion, flushing, rash, impaired renal function.

Drug Interactions: Increases risk of digoxin toxicity. Concomitant use with other antiarrhythmics increases risk of inducing hypotension. Augments pressor effects.

Pearls: Cost $$.

Causes initial rise in norepinephrine levels, which may lead to increases in BP, HR, and arrhythmias.

Pregnancy category not established.

Bretylol: see BRETYLIUM

Brevibloc: *see* **ESMOLOL**

BROMOCRIPTINE MESYLATE (Parlodel)

Dose: For Parkinson's disease, 1.25 mg (half of a 2.5 mg "Snap-Tab") PO bid with meals initially; may increase total daily dose by 2.5 mg (i.e., bid dose by 1.25 mg) every 14–28 days; max, 50 mg bid given with meals.

Preparations: 2.5 mg scored "SnapTabs"; 5 mg capsules.

Actions: Ergot derivative with potent agonistic activity against postsynaptic dopamine receptors; used to treat Parkinson's disease and other disorders (including pituitary adenoma, neuroleptic malignant syndrome, amenorrhea, galactorrhea, and female infertility). Like dopamine, inhibits pituitary secretion of prolactin.

Clearance: Metabolized via liver.
  No change in dosage needed in impaired renal function.

Side Effects: Nausea, abnormal involuntary movements, vomiting, dizziness or orthostatic hypotension, hallucinations, confusion, drowsiness, "on-off" phenomenon, ataxia, insomnia, depression, abdominal discomfort, shortness of breath, first-dose hypotensive effect.

Drug Interactions: Concomitant use with antihypertensive agents increases risk of hypotension. Dopamine antagonists (phenothiazines, haloperidol, etc.) decrease its therapeutic effect.

Cautions: Contraindicated in uncontrolled hypertension (will occasionally substantially increase BP), in toxemia of pregnancy, and in patients sensitive to ergot alkaloids.

Pearls: Cost $$$$ (5 mg ≈$200 retail/100 tablets).
  Should not be used by nursing mothers (prevents lactation).

Bronkometer: *see* **ISOETHARINE**

Bronkosol: *see* **ISOETHARINE**

BUMETANIDE (Bumex)

Dose: Route dependent.
PO: 0.5–2.0 mg qd.
IV: 0.5–1.0 mg over 1–2 min; may repeat q2–3h. Max, 10 mg daily.

Preparations: 0.5, 1.0, and 2.0 mg tablets; 0.25 mg/mL injection.

Actions: Potent loop diuretic that inhibits sodium reabsorption in the ascending loop of Henle; used as a diuretic, often in patients responsive only to high-dose Lasix.

Clearance: 81% excreted in urine, 45% in unchanged form.
No change in dosage needed in impaired renal function.

Side Effects: Profound water loss and electrolyte depletion, reductions in PO_4, K^+, and Cl^-, ototoxity (but less than with the equally effective amount of furosemide).

Cautions: Contraindicated in anuria, hepatic coma, severe electrolyte depletion, and in patients taking aminoglycosides (increases risk of ototoxicity).
Patients allergic to sulfonamides may show cross-hypersensitivity.

Pearls: Cost $$$ (2 mg $\approx$$70/100 tablets); no generic form available.
1 mg Bumex is approximately as effective as 40 mg furosemide.
Can be given IM if necessary.
Patients allergic to furosemide may lack cross-sensitivity.
Pregnancy category C.

Bumex: see BUMETANIDE

BUPROPION (Wellbutrin)

Dose: Initial, 100 mg PO bid; after 3 days may increase to 100 mg PO tid. If needed, may increase after several weeks to 100–150 mg PO tid (allow at least 4–5 h between doses). Maximum single dose, 150 mg.

Preparations: 75 and 100 mg tablets.

Actions: Monocyclic agent, unrelated to other antidepressants, that may act by inhibiting dopamine uptake; used to treat depression. Unlike tricyclics, minimally inhibits norepinephrine and serotonin reuptake.

Clearance: Extensively metabolized; some metabolites are active; renal excretion may play an important role in their clearance.

Studies in patients with cirrhosis show that metabolites accumulate at 2–3 times the levels in normal patients, so reducing the dosage in liver disease is probably advisable.

Side Effects: Agitation, restlessness, tremor, anxiety, insomnia, neuropsychiatric signs and symptoms, constipation, frequent weight loss, seizures.

Drug Interactions: L-Dopa increases its side effects.

Cautions: Use with extreme caution in patients predisposed to seizures or taking medications that lower the seizure threshold.

Use with great caution in patients who are being withdrawn from benzodiazepines or had them discontinued recently.

Pearls: Cost $$$$ (≈$2.10/d retail).

Risk of seizures is approximately 0.4% at doses up to 450 mg daily and increases substantially at higher dosages.

Its potential advantages over other antidepressants include lack of autonomic and cardiovascular effects, sedation, or weight gain.

Pregnancy category B.

BuSpar: see BUSPIRONE

BUSPIRONE (BuSpar)

Dose: Initial, 5 mg PO q8h; may increase total daily dose (*not* tid dose) by 5 mg every 2–3 days; max, 20 mg PO q8h.

Preparations: 5 and 10 mg tablets.

Actions: Anxiolytic, unrelated to benzodiazepines or barbiturates, that may act on 5-hydroxytryptophan; used to treat anxiety disorders.

Clearance: Metabolized primarily via liver.

One source recommends against giving to patients with renal impairment, but others claim no change in dosage is necessary.

Side Effects: Dizziness, light-headedness, nausea, headache, nervousness, restlessness.

Drug Interactions: Raises serum level of haloperidol. Greatly increases BP when given with MAOI.

Cautions: Contraindicated in patients receiving MAOI.

Pearls: Cost $$$$ (10 mg ≈$90 retail/100 tablets).

Should not be taken prn.

Usually is less sedating than other anxiolytics.

More effective in patients who have not previously taken benzodiazepines.

Maximum effect may take weeks to achieve.

Signs and symptoms of overdose include nausea and vomiting, dizziness, drowsiness, miosis, and GI distress.

Pregnancy category B.

BUSULFAN (Myleran)

Dose: Induction, 4–8 mg PO daily; after induction, a maintenance dose of 1–3 mg PO daily is sometimes used.

Preparations: 2 mg scored tablets.

Actions: Alkylating agent, nonspecific for cell cycle phase; used to treat neoplastic disease.

Clearance: Metabolized via liver.

Reduce dosage in ESRD (give 50% of normal dose); no change in dosage needed for milder renal impairment.

Supplemental dose not required after HD.

Side Effects: Myelosuppression, rare pulmonary fibrosis, hyperpigmentation, hyperuricemia. Prolonged use can cause adrenal insufficiency and suppression of testicular and ovarian function.

Pearls: Cost $$$ ($1/tablet wholesale).

Myelosuppression is the dose-limiting toxicity.

WBC and platelet nadirs occur 14–21 days after pulse dosing. Follow CBC.

Pulmonary fibrosis ("busulfan lung") is a rare but important side effect that usually occurs after months to years of prolonged treatment.

Pregnancy category D.

Calan: see VERAPAMIL

CALCIUM CARBONATE (Os-Cal; see also Rolaids, Tums)

Dose: 250–500 mg PO tid.

Preparations: 250 and 500 mg tablets.

Pearls: Cost $ (500 mg generic ≈$5 retail/100 tablets, Os-Cal ≈$8 retail/60 tablets).

CALCIUM CHLORIDE

Dose: (1) 2–4 mg/kg of 10% solution IV; (2) 1 amp (13.6 mEq) of a pre-mixed 10% solution IV.

Actions: Calcium supplement that can be used during cardiac arrests or to reverse the peripheral-dilating properties of the calcium antagonists.

Pearls: In emergency situations, the use of calcium chloride is preferred over other calcium supplements (such as calcium gluconate).

Capoten: see CAPTOPRIL

Capozide (CAPTOPRIL + HYDROCHLOROTHIAZIDE)

Dose: 1 tablet PO bid–tid 1 h before meals.

Preparations: Tablets containing 25 mg captopril with 15 or 25 mg hydrochlorothiazide, 50 mg captopril with 15 or 25 mg hydrochlorothiazide.

Actions: Drug that combines vasodilating and K^+-sparing properties of ACE inhibitor captopril with diuretic action of hydrochlorothiazide; used to treat hypertension.

Cautions: Contraindicated during second and third trimesters of pregnancy (because of captopril component).

Pearls: Cost $$$–$$$$ (≈$1.80/d retail).

BP-lowering action of ACE inhibitors is often strongly enhanced in fluid-depleted patients, which may increase risk of a hypotensive response.

Pregnancy category D.

CAPSAICIN cream (Axsain, Zostrix)

Dose: Apply to affected areas tid–qid.

Preparations: Axsain: 1.0 and 2.0 oz tubes containing 0.075% capsaicin; Zostrix: 1.5 and 3.0 oz tubes containing 0.025% capsaicin.

Actions: Topical analgesic that may inhibit synthesis, transport, and release of substance P, a neurotransmitter of pain; used to treat pain associated with arthritis and neuralgias.

Side Effects: Transient burning sensation at application site (caused by initial release of substance P).

Pearls: Cost $$$–$$$$ (2.0 oz tube Axsain ≈$60 retail; 1.5 oz tube Zostrix ≈$25 retail).

Inform patients that they may experience a burning sensation for the first several days of use.

Warn patients to wash hands immediately after applying cream, not to apply cream to wounds or damaged skin, and to avoid contact with eyes.

Manufacturer states that optimal benefit may take 4–6 weeks to achieve, but most patients should notice some relief of symptoms by 1–2 weeks.

Preparations of this type have a substantial placebo effect, but there appears to be at least some additional benefit from using capsaicin.

CAPTOPRIL (Capoten; *see also* Capozide)

Dose: Initial test dose, 6.25 or 12.5 mg; usual, 25–50 mg bid–tid (increase stepwise).

Preparations: 12.5, 25, 50, and 100 mg tablets.

Actions: ACE inhibitor that promotes peripheral dilatation; used to treat hypertension and CHF.

Clearance: Metabolized via liver; renal excreted.

Slightly decrease dosage or moderately increase dosing interval in impaired renal function.

One source suggests that dosage should probably be reduced in liver disease.

Supplemental dose suggested after HD.

Side Effects: Characteristic nonproductive cough (especially in women), hypotension, neutropenia (increased incidence in patients with chronic renal failure or collagen vascular disease), proteinuria, elevated BUN and creatinine, rash, dysgeusia, angioedema, laryngeal edema, cholestatic jaundice, hyperkalemia (especially in patients with impaired renal function or taking K^+-sparing drugs or K^+ supplements).

Cautions: Contraindicated during second and third trimesters of pregnancy and in patients with significant aortic stenosis or hyperkalemia.

Patients should almost never be given both an ACE inhibitor and a K^+ supplement, unless clearly indicated by serial serum K^+ testing.

Pearls: Cost $$$ ($\approx$$1.50/d retail).

Risk of hypotension is increased in volume- or NaCl-restricted patients.

Periodically check CBC, BUN, creatinine, and K^+.

Pregnancy category D.

Carafate: see SUCRALFATE

CARBACHOL eye drops

Dose: Usual, 1 or 2 drops (written "gtt") bid–tid.

Actions: Cholinergic agent that increases outflow of aqueous humor by stimulating ciliary body contraction; used to treat glaucoma.

Side Effects: Myopia with blurred vision, rare systemic effects including hypertension, tachycardia, bronchospasm.

CARBAMAZEPINE (Tegretol)

Dose: Initial, 200 mg PO bid; may increase up to 400 mg tid–qid. Usual maintenance, 400 mg PO bid–tid.

Preparations: 100 mg chewable tablets; 200 mg adult tablets; 100 mg/5 mL (1 tsp) suspension.

Actions: Anticonvulsant that probably acts by reducing poly-synaptic responses and blocking post-tetanic potentiation; used to treat seizure disorders.

Clearance: Metabolized via liver; metabolites are active.
   Slightly reduce dosage in ESRD; no change needed for milder renal impairment.
   Decrease in dosage (or at least *careful* blood level monitoring) may be needed in liver disease.
   Supplemental dose not required after HD.

Side Effects: Numerous CNS effects including drowsiness and dizziness, nausea and vomiting, diarrhea, constipation, elevated LFTs, acute urine retention, oliguria or azotemia, decreased WBCs and platelets, SIADH, pruritus and rash, numerous cardio-vascular effects.

Drug Interactions: Decreases serum levels of theophylline, war-farin, and haloperidol. Concomitant use with MAOI causes hyper-pyrexia and seizures. Phenytoin and phenobarbital decrease its serum level. Erythromycin, cimetidine, isoniazid, and calcium-channel blockers raise its serum level, increasing its potential toxicity.

Cautions: Contraindicated in patients taking MAOI or with his-tory of hypersensitivity to any tricyclic.

Pearls: Cost $$$ ($\approx$$1.50/d retail).
   Abrupt discontinuance may precipitate seizures.
   Usual therapeutic level is 4–12 μg/mL.
   Signs and symptoms of overdose include respiratory depression, convulsions, coma, tremor, arrhythmia, marked fluctuations in BP, and marked tachycardia.
   Pregnancy category C.

CARBIDOPA: see Sinemet

CARBOPLATIN (Paraplatin)

Dose: Average, 400 mg/m^2 IV.

Actions: Platinum analog that cross-links DNA molcules; used to treat malignancies.

Clearance: Significant renal excretion because of low protein binding.
Reduce dosage in impaired renal function.
No change in dosage needed for liver disease.

Side Effects: Myelosuppression, rare anaphylactoid reaction, dose-related nausea and vomiting.

Pearls: Cost $$$ (150 mg ≈$200 wholesale).
A relatively new agent with several advantages over the similar cisplatin: less nephrotoxicity, nausea and vomiting; minimal oto-toxicity, neurotoxicity, and magnesium wasting. Has greater myelosuppression, principally of platelets than cisplatin.
Pregnancy category D.

Cardene: see NICARDIPINE

Cardizem: see DILTIAZEM [IV], DILTIAZEM [PO]

Cardura: see DOXAZOSIN

CARISOPRODOL (Soma)

Dose: 350 mg PO qid; give last dose qhs.

Preparations: 350 mg tablets.

Actions: Centrally acting muscle relaxant that blocks interneuronal activity in the descending reticular formation and spinal cord in animals; used to treat muscle spasm.

Clearance: Metabolized via liver; renal excreted.
Manufacturer suggests caution in administering to patients with liver or kidney disease.

Side Effects: Drowsiness and other CNS effects, postural hypotension.

Pearls: Cost: generic $$, Soma $$$$ (generic ≈$0.60/d retail, Soma ≈$4.50/d retail).
Pregnancy category not established.

CASANTHRANOL: see Peri-Colace

Catapres: see CLONIDINE

Ceclor: see CEFACLOR

CEFACLOR (Ceclor)

Dose: 250–500 mg PO q8h without regard to meals.

Preparations: 250 and 500 mg tablets; 125 mg/5 mL (1 tsp) and 250 mg/mL suspensions.

Actions: Bactericidal second-generation cephalosporin that inhibits cell wall synthesis. Good gram (+) coverage including strep and most staph (but *not* enterococci or MRSA); some gram (−) coverage including *E. coli, Klebsiella, Proteus,* and β-lactamase–producing *H. influenzae* (though hospital-acquired gram (−) organisms are usually resistant); poor anaerobic coverage.

Clearance: Primarily renal excreted.
Slightly reduce dosage in impaired renal function.
No change in dosage needed for liver disease.
Supplemental dose suggested after HD or PD.

Side Effects: Mild decrease in WBCs, elevated LFTs, (+) Coombs' reaction, GI upset, eosinophilia, rash.

Cautions: Use with caution in patients with penicillin allergy.

Pearls: Cost $$$ (≈$60/wk retail). See under Penicillin for a comparison of weekly costs for brand-name and generic oral antibiotics.
Pregnancy category B.

CEFADROXIL (Duricef)

Dose: 1–2 g PO daily given in 1 or 2 divided doses with meals.

Preparations: 500 mg and 1 g tablets; 50 and 100 mL bottles of orange-pineapple flavored oral suspension, available in concentrations of 125, 250, and 500 mg/5 mL (1 tsp).

Actions: Semisynthetic bactericidal cephalosporin that inhibits cell wall synthesis. Good gram (+) coverage including strep and many staph (but *not* enterococci or MRSA); some gram (−) coverage (but not *P. aeruginosa*, β-lactamase–producing *H. influenzae*, or hospital-acquired organisms); poor anaerobic coverage.

Clearance: Excreted unchanged in urine.
Slightly to moderately increase dosing interval in impaired renal function.

Side Effects: Allergic reactions, GI side effects, pseudomembranous colitis.

Cautions: Use with caution in penicillin allergy.

Pearls: Cost $$$ (≈$50/wk retail).
Should be taken with meals to decrease GI side effects.
Pregnancy category B.

CEFAMANDOLE (Mandol)

Dose: 500 mg–2 g IM or IV q4–6h.

Preparations: 500 mg, 1 g, and 2 g vials for injection.

Actions: Bactericidal second-generation cephalosporin that inhibits cell wall synthesis. Good gram (+) coverage (but *not* MRSA or enterococci); moderate gram (−) coverage including β-lactamase–producing organisms (but *not P. aeruginosa* and many nosocomial infections); poor anaerobic coverage.

Clearance: Renal excreted.
Slightly to moderately increase dosing interval, reduce dosage, or both, in impaired renal function.
No change in dosage needed for liver disease.
Supplemental dose suggested after HD.

Side Effects: Hypersensitivity reactions.

Drug Interactions: Probenecid raises its serum level. Rare Antabuse-like reaction with alcohol. Concomitant use with aminoglycosides increases risk of nephrotoxicity.

Cautions: Use with caution in patients with penicillin allergy.

Pearls: Cost $$$ (≈$40/d wholesale).
Pregnancy category B.

CEFAZOLIN (Ancef, Kefzol)

Dose: Infection dependent.
Mild infection: 250–500 mg IM or IV q8h.
Moderate to severe infection: 500–1000 mg IM or IV q6–8h.
Life-threatening infection: 1000–1500 mg IM or IV q6h.

Preparations: 250 and 500 mg vials for injection; Kefzol is also available in 1 and 10 g vials.

Actions: Bactericidal first-generation cephalosporin that inhibits cell wall synthesis. Good gram (+) coverage including *S. aureus* and strep (but *not* MRSA or enterococci); some gram (−) coverage including *E. coli, Klebsiella,* and *Proteus* (hospital-acquired gram (−) organisms are usually resistant); poor anaerobic coverage.

Clearance: Primarily renal excreted.
Moderately reduce dosage in impaired renal function.
No change in dosage needed for liver disease.
Supplemental dose suggested after HD but not after PD.

Side Effects: Elevated LFTs, GI distress, pseudomembranous colitis.

Drug Interactions: Concomitant use with aminoglycosides increases risk of nephrotoxicity. Probenecid and sulfinpyrazone may raise its serum level.

Cautions: Use with caution in patients with penicillin allergy.

Pearls: Cost $ (≈$11/d wholesale).
Well tolerated IM.
Pregnancy category B.

CEFIXIME (Suprax)

Dose: 200 mg PO q12h or 400 mg PO qd without regard to meals.

Preparations: 200 and 400 mg scored tablets; 50 and 100 mL bottles containing powder for strawberry-flavored oral suspension that contains 100 mg/5 mL (1 tsp) when reconstituted.

Actions: Semisynthetic bactericidal cephalosporin that inhibits cell wall synthesis. Poor gram (+) coverage with variable coverage for strep (but *not* staph or enterococci); good gram (−) coverage (but *not P. aeruginosa*); poor anaerobic coverage.

Clearance: 50% of absorbed dose is excreted unchanged in the urine.
Slightly reduce dosage in impaired renal function.
Is not significantly removed by HD or PD.

Side Effects: Diarrhea, nausea, dyspepsia, abdominal pain, flatulence.

Cautions: Use with caution in patients with penicillin allergy.

Pearls: Cost $$$$ (>$5/d retail!).
Pregnancy category B.

Cefizox: see CEFTIZOXIME

Cefobid: see CEFOPERAZONE

CEFOPERAZONE (Cefobid)

Dose: 1–2 g IM or IV q12h.

Preparations: 1 and 2 g vials.

Actions: Bactericidal third-generation cephalosporin that inhibits cell wall synthesis. Excellent gram (−) coverage including *P. aeruginosa;* some gram (+) coverage; variable *B. fragilis* coverage.

Clearance: Excreted in bile.
No change in dosage needed in impaired renal function.
Serum $t_{1/2}$ is increased 2–4 times in patients with significant liver disease.

Pearls: Cost $$ (≈$30/d wholesale).
Pregnancy category B.

Cefotan: see CEFOTETAN

CEFOTAXIME (Claforan)

Dose: Infection dependent.

Usual, 1–2 g IM or IV q8–12h.

Life-threatening infection: Up to 2 g IV q4h; max, 12 g in 24 h.

Preparations: 1 and 2 g vials for injection.

Actions: Bactericidal third-generation cephalosporin that inhibits cell wall synthesis. Some gram (+) coverage (but *not* MRSA or enterococci); excellent gram (−) coverage (but *not P. aeruginosa*); some anaerobes including some *B. fragilis.*

Clearance: Metabolized via liver; renal excreted; metabolites are active in ESRD.

Moderately increase dosing interval in impaired renal function.

May need to adjust dosing interval in severe liver disease.

Supplemental dose suggested after HD but not after PD.

Side Effects: Local pain at IM site or phlebitis at IV site, hypersensitivity reaction, GI distress, nausea and vomiting, elevated LFTs, eosinophilia, (+) Coombs' reaction, pseudomembranous colitis.

Drug Interactions: Concomitant use with aminoglycosides increases risk of nephrotoxicity.

Cautions: Use with caution in patients with penicillin allergy.

Pearls: Cost $$1/2 (≈$40/d wholesale).

Pregnancy category B.

CEFOTETAN (Cefotan)

Dose: 1–3 g IM or IV q12h.

Preparations: 1 and 2 g vials for injection.

Actions: Bactericidal second-generation cephalosporin that inhibits cell wall synthesis. Some gram (+) coverage (but *not* MRSA or enterococci); excellent gram (−) coverage including β-lactamase–producing organisms (but *not P. aeruginosa;*) good anaerobic coverage including *B. fragilis.*

Clearance: Primarily renal excreted.
   Moderately reduce dosage in impaired renal function.
   No change in dosage needed for liver disease.
   Supplemental dose suggested after HD but not PD.

Side Effects: Diarrhea, nausea, rash, hypersensitivity reaction.

Drug Interactions: Disulfiram-like reaction with alcohol. Concomitant use with aminoglycosides increases risk of nephrotoxicity.

Cautions: Use with caution in patients with penicillin allergy.

Pearls: Cost $$ (≈$40/d wholesale).
   Pregnancy category B.

CEFOXITIN (Mefoxin)

Dose: 1–2 g IV q8–12h; may be given IM.

Preparations: 1 and 2 g vials for injection.

Actions: Bactericidal second-generation cephalosporin that inhibits cell wall synthesis. Some gram (+) coverage (but *not* enterococci); good gram (−) coverage including *E. coli, Proteus, Klebsiella,* and *H. influenzae* (but *not P. aeruginosa*); excellent anaerobic coverage (including *B. fragilis*).

Clearance: Renal excreted.
   Moderately increase dosing interval in impaired renal function.
   No change in dosage required for liver disease.
   Supplemental dose suggested after HD but not after PD.

Side Effects: Rash, eosinophilia, pruritus, fever, (+) Coombs' reaction, mild decrease in WBCs, elevated LFTs.

Drug Interactions: Concomitant use with aminoglycosides may increase risk of nephrotoxicity. Probenecid and sulfinpyrazone may raise its serum level.

Cautions: Use with caution in patients with penicillin allergy.

Pearls: Cost $$ (≈$30/d wholesale).
   Can *falsely* raise measured serum creatinine levels.
   Pregnancy category B.

CEFTAZIDIME (Fortaz, Tazicef, Tazidime)

Dose: 1–2 g IM or IV q8–12h; usual, 1 g IV q8h.

Preparations: 0.5, 1, and 2 g vials for injection.

Actions: Bactericidal third-generation cephalosporin that inhibits cell wall synthesis. Excellent gram (−) coverage, particularly for *P. aeruginosa;* poor gram (+) or anaerobic coverage.

Clearance: Primarily renal excreted.
  Markedly increase dosing interval in impaired renal function.
  No change in dosage needed for liver disease.
  Supplemental dose suggested after HD or PD.

Side Effects: Local phlebitis, rash, eosinophilia, elevated LFTs, increased platelets, (+) Coombs' reaction.

Drug Interactions: Concomitant use with aminoglycosides may increase risk of nephrotoxicity.

Cautions: Use with caution in patients with penicillin allergy.

Pearls: Cost $$$ (≈$45/d wholesale).
  (+) CSF penetration in meningeal inflammation.
  Pregnancy category B.

Ceftin: see CEFUROXIME

CEFTIZOXIME (Cefizox)

Dose: 1–2 g IV q8–12h; usual, 1 g IV q8h.

Preparations: 1 and 2 g vials for injection.

Actions: Bactericidal third-generation cephalosporin that inhibits cell wall synthesis. Excellent gram (−) coverage (but *not Pseudomonas*); some gram (+) coverage including *S. aureus* and strep (but *not* MRSA or enterococci); some anaerobic coverage (some strains of *B. fragilis* are resistant).

Clearance: Renal excreted.
  Markedly increase dosing interval in impaired renal function.
  No change in dosage needed for liver disease.
  Supplemental dose suggested after HD.

Side Effects: Local phlebitis, elevated LFTs, rash, eosinophilia, (+) Coombs' reaction.

Drug Interactions: Concomitant use with aminoglycosides may increase risk of nephrotoxicity. Probenecid may raise its serum level.

Cautions: Use with caution in patients with penicillin allergy.

Pearls: Cost $$ ($\approx$$30/d wholesale).
(+) CSF penetration in meningeal inflammation.
Pregnancy category B.

CEFTRIAXONE (Rocephin)

Dose: Disease dependent.
Systemic nongonococcal infection: 1–2 g IM or IV q12–24h; usually given q24h (because of long $t_{1/2}$) except in meningitis, for which the dosage may be 2 g q12h.
Nonsystemic gonococcal infection: Single dose of 250 mg IM.

Preparations: 0.25, 0.5, 1, and 2 g vials for injection.

Actions: Bactericidal third-generation cephalosporin that inhibits cell wall synthesis. Excellent gram (−) coverage (but *not Pseudomonas*); some gram (+) coverage including *S. aureus* and strep (but *not* MRSA, enterococci, or *Listeria*); some anaerobic coverage (some strains of *B. fragilis* are resistant).

Clearance: Secreted in bile; renal excreted (60%).
Slightly increase dosing interval in ESRD; no change needed for milder renal impairment.
Follow patients carefully for severe liver disease.
Give maximum of 2 g daily in patients with *both* hepatic and renal failure.
Supplemental dose not required after HD or PD.

Side Effects: Local phlebitis, rash, eosinophilia, reduced WBCs, increased platelets, elevated LFTs, increased BUN and creatinine, diarrhea, possible cholestatic impairment.

Cautions: Use with caution in patients with penicillin allergy.

Pearls: Cost $$1/2 ($\approx$$30/d wholesale).
($+$) CSF penetration in meningeal inflammation.
Consider following serum levels in patients with impaired renal function.
Can exacerbate vitamin K deficiency in predisposed patients.
If used for empiric coverage of meningitis in elderly or debilitated patients, many sources now recommend also using ampicillin to cover for *Listeria* (which ceftriaxone does not cover).
Pregnancy category B.

CEFUROXIME (PO = Ceftin; IV = Kefurox, Zinacef)

Dose: Route dependent.
PO: 125–500 mg q12h without regard to meals.
IV: 750–1500 mg q8h.

Preparations: 125, 250, and 500 mg tablets of Ceftin; 0.25, 0.5, 1, and 10 g vials for injection of Kefurox; 0.75 and 1.5 g vials for injection of Zinacef.

Actions: Bactericidal second-generation cephalosporin that inhibits cell wall synthesis. Good gram ($-$) coverage including β-lactamase–producing organisms (but *not P. aeruginosa*); good gram ($+$) coverage including *S. aureus* and strep (but *not* enterococci or MRSA); *not* most *B. fragilis*.

Clearance: Renal excreted.
Markedly reduce dosage in impaired renal function.
Supplemental dose suggested after HD but not after PD.

Side Effects: Phlebitis, eosinophilia, rare elevated LFTs, reduced hematocrit, rare decrease in WBCs or ($+$) Coombs' reaction.

Drug Interactions: Concomitant use with aminoglycosides may increase risk of nephrotoxicity. Probenecid may raise its serum level.

Cautions: Use with caution in patients with penicillin allergy.

Pearls: Cost $$$ (PO $\approx$$45/wk retail; IV $\approx$$20–$40/d wholesale). See under Penicillin for a comparison of weekly costs for brand-name and generic oral antibiotics.
Clinically ineffective in meningitis.
Pregnancy category B.

CEPHALEXIN (Keflex, Keftab)

Dose: 250–500 mg PO qid without regard to meals.

Preparations: 250 and 500 mg tablets; 125 and 250 mg/5 mL (1 tsp) suspensions.

Actions: Bactericidal first-generation cephalosporin that inhibits cell wall synthesis. Good gram (+) coverage including *S. aureus* and strep (but *not* MRSA or enterococci); some gram (−) coverage including *E. coli, Proteus,* and *Klebsiella* (but *not P. aeruginosa* or nosocomial infections); poor anaerobic coverage.

Clearance: Renal excreted, but only slightly reduce dosage in impaired renal function.
No change in dosage needed for liver disease.
Supplemental dose suggested after HD or PD.

Side Effects: GI distress, rash, eosinophilia, mild reduction in WBCs, elevated LFTs, (+) Coombs' reaction.

Cautions: Use with caution in patients with penicillin allergy.

Pearls: Cost $$$ (≈$32/wk retail). See under Penicillin for a comparison of weekly costs for brand-name and generic oral antibiotics.
Pregnancy category B.

Cerubidine: see DAUNORUBICIN

Cerumenex: see TRIETHANOLAMINE otic solution

CHARCOAL (ACTIVATED CHARCOAL)

Dose: Suggested regimens include:
(1) 20–50 g PO or via NG tube q2–6h for 24 h.
(2) 50–100 mg PO or via NG tube q4–6h for 24 h.

Preparations: Multiple size bottles; some preparations come premixed with sorbitol.

Actions: Inert substance that absorbs most drugs; used to treat drug overdose.

Pearls: Often given repeatedly with drugs that undergo hepatobiliary excretion.

Does *not* absorb alkalis, mineral acids, or $FeSO_4$.

Concomitant use with cathartics may reduce its effectiveness.

May absorb oral antidotes (i.e., Mucomyst).

CHLORAMBUCIL (Leukeran)

Dose: Initial, 4–10 mg (0.1–0.2 mg/kg) PO qd; maintenance, 2–4 mg (0.03–0.1 mg/kg) PO qd.

Give before or after meals (food reduces its bioavailability).

Preparations: 2 mg tablets.

Actions: Alkylating agent; used to treat neoplastic diseases.

Clearance: Extensively metabolized in the liver to inactive metabolites; almost no renal excretion.

Side Effects: Myelosuppression, rare pulmonary fibrosis, rare hepatotoxicity, rare seizures.

Pearls: Cost $$$.

Myelosuppression (especially of platelets) is dose-limiting toxicity.

WBC and platelet nadirs usually occur 14–21 days after treatment.

Pulmonary fibrosis is a rare side effect and usually occurs months to years after prolonged treatment.

Pregnancy category D.

CHLORAMPHENICOL (Chloromycetin)

Dose: 12.5–25 mg/kg PO q6h (50–100 mg/kg daily).

Preparations: 250 mg Chloromycetin Kapseals.

Actions: Broad-spectrum antibiotic that inhibits protein synthesis; used to treat serious gram (+) and gram (−) infections for which less potentially dangerous drugs are ineffective or contraindicated. Bacteriostatic against most organisms and bactericidal against pneumococci, *H. influenzae,* and meningococci. Particularly useful in meningitis and in *Salmonella typhi* and *H. influenzae* infection.

Clearance: 70–90% metabolized in the liver to inactive metabolites.

May need to reduce dosage in severe renal dysfunction.

Decrease dosage in liver disease.

Supplemental dose suggested after HD but not after PD.

Side Effects: Dose-related reversible bone marrow suppression, aplastic anemia (rare but irreversible), nausea and vomiting, headache, mild depression, confusion and delirium, hypersensitivity reactions including fever, rash, angioedema, urticaria, and anaphylaxis.

Cautions: May cause "gray syndrome" in children born to pregnant women given this drug.

Pearls: Cost $$ (≈$16/d retail).

Excellent CSF penetration.

Risk of aplastic anemia, listed in various sources as 1/24,200 to 1/100,000, is not dose related and occurs weeks to months after therapy.

Should generally not be used in pregnant patients.

CHLORDIAZEPOXIDE (Librium)

Dose: Disease dependent.

Anxiety: 5–25 mg PO tid–qid (in elderly patients give 5 mg bid–qid).

Alcohol withdrawal: Highly individualized by physician and variable by patient; one suggested regimen is 50–100 mg IM or IV, repeated in 2–4 h if necessary.

Preparations: 5, 10, and 25 mg capsules; 100 mg ampules for injection.

Actions: Benzodiazepine with antianxiety, sedative, and muscle-relaxant properties; used to treat anxiety or alcohol withdrawal.

Clearance: Metabolized in the liver; active metabolites are renal excreted.

Slightly decrease dosage in impaired renal function.

Reduce dosage in liver disease (though the extent of drug accumulation may not correlate with sedative effects).

Supplemental dose not required after HD.

Side Effects: Drowsiness, ataxia, confusion.

Cautions: Should not be used in early pregnancy or in potentially pregnant patients.

Pearls: Cost: generic $, Librium $$$ (100 tablets retail: 10 mg generic ≈$10, 10 mg Librium ≈$45, 25 mg generic ≈$10, 25 mg Librium ≈$75).

Relatively long $t_{1/2}$ may lead to accumulation; some physicians prefer Ativan for treatment of alcohol withdrawal.

Should be avoided during early pregnancy.

Chloromycetin: see CHLORAMPHENICOL

CHLOROTHIAZIDE (Diuril)

Dose: 0.5–1.0 g qd–bid PO or IV.

Preparations: 250 and 500 mg tablets; 250 mg/5 mL (1 tsp) suspension; 0.5 g vials.

Actions: Thiazide diuretic that affects electrolyte reabsorption in renal tubules; used to treat hypertension.

Clearance: Primarily renal excreted. Avoid in ESRD.

Side Effects: Azotemia, hyponatremia, hypochloremic alkalosis, hypokalemia, hypotension, hyperuricemia, elevated cholesterol and triglycerides.

Drug Interactions: May increase or decrease insulin requirements.

Cautions: Patients allergic to sulfa drugs may show cross-sensitivity.

Pearls: Cost $ (500 mg PO: generic ≈$0.10/d retail, Diuril ≈$0.20/d retail).

Onset of action: PO <2 h with peak at 4 h and duration 6–12 h; IV, 15 min with peak at 30 min.

May deleteriously alter lipid and glucose metabolism.

Pregnancy category not established.

CHLORPHENIRAMINE (Chlor-Trimeton; *see also* Allerest, Contac)

Dose: Use dependent.
   Chronic allergy (hay fever, etc.): 4 mg PO q4–6h, or 8 mg SR tablet q8h, or 12 mg SR tablet q12h. Some sources suggest beginning therapy at lower doses and gradually increasing to these levels.
   Acute allergic reaction: 12 mg PO in 1–3 divided doses.

Preparations: 4 mg tablets; 8 and 12 mg sustained-release tablets; 4 oz syrup containing 2 mg/5 mL (1 tsp).

Actions: Antihistamine with anticholinergic and sedative effects; used to treat allergic reactions and allergic rhinitis.

Pearls: When taken for chronic allergies, instruct patients to use regularly and not intermittently or prn.
   Pregnancy category B.

CHLORPROMAZINE (Thorazine)

Dose: Disease and route dependent.
   Nausea and vomiting: PO, 10–25 mg q4–6h of regular tablets or SR capsules prn. IM, 25 mg initially; if no hypotension occurs, may give 25–50 mg q3–4h prn. PR, 50–100 mg suppository q6–8h prn.
   Acute psychotic disorder: 25 mg IM; if necessary, may give additional 25–50 mg IM 1 h later.
   Intractable hiccups: 25–50 mg PO tid–qid; if symptoms persist for 2–3 days, may give 25–50 mg IM.

Preparations: 10, 25, 50, 100, and 200 mg tablets; 30, 75, 150, 200, and 300 mg sustained-release capsules; 10 mg/5 mL (1 tsp) syrup; 30 mg/mL concentrate; 25 and 100 mg suppositories; 25 mg/mL injection.

Actions: Phenothiazine; used to treat (1) nausea and vomiting, (2) psychotic disorders, (3) intractable hiccups.

Clearance: Metabolized via liver.

No change in dosage needed for impaired renal function.

Consider reducing dosage in liver disease (patients have increased CNS sensitivity to phenothiazines).

Supplemental dose not required after HD or PD.

Side Effects: CNS (drowsiness, dizziness, insomnia, fatigue, extrapyramidal reactions, tardive dyskinesia, dystonia, akathisia, rigidity, tremor, neuroleptic malignant syndrome), peripheral anticholinergic effects (blurred vision, urine retention, constipation, etc.), disulfiram-like reaction with alcohol, orthostatic hypotension, elevated LFTs and cholestatic jaundice, anorexia, muscle weakness, reduced CBC.

Drug Interactions: Antacids inhibit its absorption. Barbiturates can reduce its effectiveness. Potentiates CNS depressant effects of other CNS depressants. Concomitant use with propranolol can raise serum levels of both drugs. Can shorten PT in patients taking warfarin.

Cautions: Use with caution in patients with history of seizures (can lower the convulsive threshold).

Pearls: Cost: generic $, Thorazine $$$ (100 tablets retail: 50 mg generic ≈$10, 50 mg Thorazine ≈$60).

Pregnancy category not established.

CHLORPROPAMIDE (Diabinese)

Dose: Initial, 250 mg PO qd (100 or 125 mg PO qd in elderly patients); usual max, 500 mg PO qd.

Preparations: 100 and 250 mg tablets.

Actions: Oral hypoglycemic agent of the sulfonylurea class; used to treat non-insulin-dependent diabetes.

Clearance: Renal excreted.

Do not use if GFR <50 mL/min.

Supplemental dose not required after PD.

Side Effects: Hypoglycemia, diarrhea, vomiting, anorexia, rash, Antabuse-like reaction with alcohol, rare cholestatic jaundice or reduced CBC.

Drug Interactions: Increased hypoglycemia with concomitant use of other sulfonylureas, insulin, ASA, NSAID, sulfonamides, warfarin, MAOI, or β-blockers. Increased hyperglycemia when used with diuretics, steroids, thyroid hormone, phenothiazines, phenytoin, nicotinic acid, sympathomimetic drugs, calcium-channel blockers, or isoniazid.

Pearls: Cost: generic $, Diabinese $$ (250 mg: generic ≈$0.15/d retail, Diabinese ≈$0.50/d retail).
Duration of action 40–72 h.
Hypoglycemia is increased in elderly, debilitated, or malnourished patients; in renal, hepatic, adrenal, or pituitary impairment; with alcohol; and with severe or prolonged exercise.
Pregnancy category C.

Chlor-Trimeton: see CHLORPHENIRAMINE

CHOLESTYRAMINE (Cholybar, Questran)

Dose: 1 packet, 1 scoop, or 1 Cholybar (each containing 4 g of resin) 1–6 times daily PO.

Preparations: Cartons of 60 packets (each 9 g packet contains 4 g cholestyramine resin); cans containing 378 g Questran; cartons containing 25 caramel- or raspberry-flavored Cholybars.

Actions: Bile acid sequestrant; used to treat hypercholesterolemia.

Clearance: Not absorbed.
No change in dosage needed for impaired renal function.

Side Effects: Frequent constipation, flatulence, reduced absorption of vitamins A, D, E, and K. May prolong PT.

Drug Interactions: Decreases intestinal absorption of digoxin, penicillin, phenobarbital, propranolol, thyroid supplements, warfarin, and fat-soluble vitamins.

Cautions: Contraindicated in biliary obstruction.

Pearls: Cost $$$$ (1 packet ≈$1 retail, 1 Cholybar ≈$1.40 retail).

Rarely tolerated more than bid–tid.

Compliance may be significantly affected by its powdery taste.

Instruct patients to take other oral medications 1 h before or 4–6 h after each dose.

Pregnancy category not designated, but patients should be watched for decreased absorption of fat-soluble vitamins.

Cholybar: see CHOLESTYRAMINE

CILASTATIN: see Primaxin

CIMETIDINE (Tagamet)

Dose: Acute therapy: 300 mg PO or IV qid, or 400 mg PO bid, or 800 mg PO qhs; maintenance: 400 mg PO qhs.

Preparations: 200, 300, 400, and 800 mg tablets; 300 mg/5 mL (1 tsp) liquid; 300 mg/2 mL injection.

Actions: H_2-blocker; used to treat peptic ulcer disease.

Clearance: Metabolized via liver; renal excreted.
   Slightly reduce dosage in impaired renal function.
   No change in dosage needed for liver failure.
   Supplemental dose not required after HD or PD.

Side Effects: Elevated LFTs, diarrhea, confusion, very rare decrease in WBCs or platelets, gynecomastia, rash, reduced sperm count.

Drug Interactions: Raises serum levels of phenytoin, lidocaine, propranolol, quinidine, nifedipine, procainamide, metoprolol, and aminophylline. Prolongs PT in patients taking warfarin. Magnesium and aluminum hydroxide antacids (such as Maalox and Mylanta) reduce its bioavailability and should be given at least 2 h apart from it.

Pearls: Cost $$$ (PO ≈$1/tablet retail, IV ≈$15/d wholesale).
   Pregnancy category not established.

Cipro: see CIPROFLOXACIN

CIPROFLOXACIN (Cipro)

Dose: Route dependent.
PO: 250–750 mg bid without regard to meals (but *not* with magnesium- or aluminum-containing antacids); usual, 500 mg bid.
IV: 200–400 mg q12h.

Preparations: 250, 500, and 750 mg tablets; IV for injection.

Actions: Bactericidal synthetic broad-spectrum fluoroquinolone antibiotic that inhibits DNA gyrase. Excellent gram ($-$) coverage including *P. aeruginosa;* some gram ($+$) coverage including *S. aureus* (including resistant strains) and *S. epidermidis* (but less against strep and enterococci); *not* effective against anaerobes. Sanford's antimicrobial guide considers enterococci to be resistant to Cipro. Increasingly, problems are developing with staph isolates resistance to Cipro.

Clearance: Metabolized in liver and intestine and biliary and renally excreted.
Slightly reduce dosage or increase dosing interval in impaired renal function.
No change in dosage needed for liver disease.
Supplemental dose suggested after HD or PD.

Side Effects: GI distress, dizziness, light-headedness, CNS toxicity.

Drug Interactions: Raises serum level of theophylline. Zinc, iron, or calcium tablets reduce its absorption. Magnesium hydroxide or aluminum hydroxide antacids and sucralfate decrease its intestinal absorption.

Cautions: Avoid in patients <18 years old.

Pearls: Cost $$$ ($\approx$$43/wk retail). See under Penicillin for a comparison of weekly costs for brand-name and generic oral antibiotics.
Pregnancy category C.

Cis-P: see CISPLATIN

CISPLATIN (Cis-P)

Dose: Tumor dependent.

Actions: Antineoplastic alkylating agent; used to treat numerous malignancies.

Clearance: 27–43% renal excreted; no liver metabolism.
Do not administer if CrCl <50 mL/min.
No change in dosage needed for liver disease.
Supplemental dose suggested after HD.

Side Effects: Myelosuppression, nephrotoxicity, neuropathy, ototoxicity, anaphylactic reaction, Coombs' (+) hemolytic anemia, marked nausea and vomiting, significant electrolyte depletion (Mg^{ff}, Ca^{ff}, K^+, PO_4^+, Na^+).

Drug Interactions: Concomitant use with aminoglycosides increases risk of nephrotoxicity.

Pearls: Cost $$$ (50 mg ≈$128 wholesale).
Nephrotoxicity and peripheral neuropathy are the major dose-limiting toxicities. Nephrotoxicity usually first appears during the second week after treatment; neuropathy is directly related to cumulative dose. Usual signs include elevation of BUN, creatinine, and uric acid levels with decreased CrCl.
IV hydration and mannitol (or furosemide) are frequently used as premedication to decrease renal toxicity.
Electrolyte replacement is usually necessary during therapy.
Repeat treatment should not be given until creatinine <1.5, BUN <25, platelets >100,000, and WBCs >4000.
Audiometric testing is recommended before treatment.
Check BUN, creatinine, CrCl, Mg^{ff}, K^+, and Ca^{ff} before treatment.
Follow CBC, electrolytes, LFTs, and neurologic status.
Pregnancy category not established.

Claforan see CEFOTAXIME

CLARITHROMYCIN (Biaxin)

Dose: Disease dependent. May be given without regard to meals.

Pneumonia: 250 mg PO bid for 7–14 days.
Bronchitis: 250–500 mg PO bid for 7–14 days.
Pharyngitis or tonsillitis: 250 mg PO bid for 10 days.
Sinusitis: 500 mg PO bid for 14 days.

Preparations: 250 and 500 mg tablets.

Actions: Bactericidal macrolide antibiotic with bacterial coverage that can be thought of as a combination of erythromycin and the β-lactams. Good gram (+) coverage including *S. aureus, S. pneumoniae,* and group A strep (but *not* MRSA or enterococci); some gram (−) coverage including *H. influenzae.* Also covers *M. pneumoniae* and *M. catarrhalis (Branhamella catarrhalis).* Has been shown in vitro to cover *Legionella pneumophila.*

Clearance: Metabolized via liver; renal excreted.
Reduce dosage or increase dosing interval in impaired renal function.
No change in dosage needed for liver disease.

Side Effects: Predominantly GI, including diarrhea, nausea, abnormal taste, dyspepsia.

Drug Interactions: Raises serum levels of theophylline and possibly carbamazepine. Although not reported in clinical trials with clarithromycin, erythromycin has been reported to raise serum levels of digoxin and of drugs metabolized by the cytochrome P-450 system, and to prolong PT in patients taking warfarin.

Cautions: Contraindicated in erythromycin allergy. Should not be used in pregnant or potentially pregnant patients.

Pearls: Cost $$$ (≈$43/wk retail). See under Penicillin for a comparison of weekly costs for brand-name and generic oral antibiotics.
No cross-allergenicity in patients allergic to penicillin or cephalosporins.
Do *not* give during pregnancy.

CLAVULANATE: see Augmentin, Timentin

Clearasil: see BENZOYL PEROXIDE

Cleocin: see CLINDAMYCIN

Cleocin T: see CLINDAMYCIN PHOSPHATE

CLINDAMYCIN (Cleocin)

Dose: Disease dependent.
Systemic infection: usual, 600 mg IM or IV q8h.
Intraluminal GI tract infection: 300 mg PO qid.

Preparations: 75, 150, and 300 mg capsules; 75 mg/5 mL (1 tsp) suspension; IV for injection.

Actions: Bacteriostatic antibiotic that reversibly inhibits protein synthesis. Good gram (+) coverage (but *not* enterococci or MRSA); *no* gram (−) coverage; excellent anaerobic coverage (5% of *Bacteroides* are resistant).

Clearance: Metabolized primarily in the liver to inactive and less active metabolites.
No change in dosage needed for mild to moderate renal impairment; use with caution in severe renal disease.
No change in dosage required for mild to moderate liver dysfunction; reduce dosage in moderate to severe liver disease.
Supplemental dose not required after HD or PD.

Side Effects: Local phlebitis, GI upset, diarrhea, pseudomembranous colitis, elevated LFTs, hypersensitivity reactions.

Drug Interactions: Enhances action of nondepolarizing muscle relaxants.

Pearls: Cost $$$ (PO ≈$12/d retail, IV ≈$80/d wholesale).
(−) CSF penetration.
Has neuromuscular blocking properties that may potentiate other neuromuscular blockers.
Carries high risk of *C. difficile* diarrhea or colitis.
Pregnancy category not established.

CLINDAMYCIN PHOSPHATE topical solution, lotion, and gel (Cleocin T)

Dose: Apply thin film to affected skin bid.

Preparations: 30 mL, 60 mL, and 16 oz bottles of solution; 7.5 and 30 g tubes of gel; 60 mL plastic squeeze-bottles of lotion.

Actions: Topical antibiotic; used to treat acne vulgaris.

Side Effects: Dry skin. Diarrhea, bloody diarrhea, and colitis (including pseudomembranous colitis) can occur with topical form.

Cautions: Contraindicated in patients with history of regional enteritis, ulcerative colitis, or antibiotic-associated colitis.

Pearls: Cost $$ (30 g tube ≈$22 retail).
Pregnancy category B.

Clinoril: see SULINDAC

CLOMIPRAMINE (Anafranil)

Dose: Initial, 25 mg PO qd with food; may be gradually increased over next 2 weeks to total of 100 mg daily, given in divided doses with meals.

May gradually titrate over next several weeks to maximum of 250 mg daily given in divided doses with meals.

Once optimal dosage is reached, entire daily dose may be given qhs.

Preparations: 25, 50, and 75 mg capsules.

Actions: Tricyclic antidepressant that may inhibit serotonin reuptake; used to treat obsessive-compulsive disorders.

Clearance: Metabolized to the active metabolite desmethylclomipramine; effects of hepatic or renal disease on its elimination have not been determined.

Side Effects: Seizure, dry mouth, constipation, nausea, anorexia, dyspepsia, somnolence, tremor, dizziness, nervousness, myoclonus, modest orthostatic changes and modest tachycardia, elevated LFTs, sexual dysfunction or reduced libido (common), weight gain, visual changes, blood dyscrasias.

Cautions: Contraindicated in patients with history of hypersensitivity to tricyclics and during acute recovery period following MI.
Should not be given within 14 days of MAOI.

Pearls: Cost $$$$ (>$2/d retail).

Steady-state plasma levels may not be reached for up to 3 weeks, so allow 2–3 weeks between further dosage changes.

Pregnancy category C.

CLONAZEPAM (Klonopin; formerly Clonopin)

Dose: Initial, up to 0.5 mg PO tid; may gradually increase until seizures are controlled; max, 20 mg daily.

Preparations: 0.5, 1.0, and 2.0 mg tablets.

Actions: Benzodiazepine; used to treat petit-mal seizures.

Clearance: Metabolized via liver. No change in dosage needed for impaired renal function.

Side Effects: CNS depression, drowsiness, ataxia.

Drug Interactions: Potentiates CNS depressant effects of other CNS depressants.

Cautions: Contraindicated in liver disease or narrow-angle glaucoma.

Pearls: Cost $$$$ (1.0 mg ≈$70 retail/100 tablets).

Abrupt withdrawal can precipitate tonic-clonic seizures.

Can increase incidence or precipitate onset of tonic-clonic seizures.

Pregnancy category not established.

CLONIDINE (Catapres, Catapres-TTS)

Dose: Route dependent.

PO: Initial, 0.1 mg bid (may start lower in elderly patients); may increase by 0.1 mg daily. Usual, 0.1–0.3 mg bid. Max, 1.2 mg bid.

Catapres-TSS Patch: One TTS-1 weekly for 2 weeks, then may increase by equivalent of 0.1 mg daily each subsequent week. Max, two TTS-3 patches per week (equivalent to 0.6 mg daily).

Preparations: 0.1, 0.2, and 0.3 mg tablets; TTS-1, TTS-2, and TTS-3 patches delivering 0.1, 0.2, and 0.3 mg daily, respectively.

Actions: Centrally acting α-antagonist; used to treat hypertension.

Clearance: Metabolized via liver; renal excreted.
Slightly reduce dosage in ESRD; no change needed for milder renal impairment.
Reduce dosage in liver dysfunction.
Supplemental dose not required after HD.

Side Effects: Dry mouth, drowsiness, dizziness, constipation, sedation, weakness, fatigue, headache, parotid pain, rare depression (1%).

Drug Interactions: Tricyclics reduce its effectiveness. Increases CNS depressant effects of alcohol and other sedatives. Diminishes or reverses antihypertensive effects of β-blockers.

Cautions: May be contraindicated in pregnant patients (has known embryotoxic effects in animals).

Pearls: Cost: generic $$, Catapres tablets $$$, Catapres patch $$$ (100 tablets retail: 0.1 mg generic ≈$17, 0.1 mg Catapres ≈$45, 0.3 mg generic ≈$34, 0.3 mg Catapres ≈$100; 1 Catapres patch retail: TSS-1 ≈$7.50, TSS-3 ≈$17).
Use PO form with caution in patients who develop localized skin sensitivity from the patch.
Withdrawal reactions sometimes occur, usually if patients are taking >1.2 mg daily *or* if also taking β-blockers; to avoid withdrawal reactions, taper over 2–4 days when indicated.
Therapeutic drug levels are achieved with the patch after 2–3 days.
Pregnancy category not established, but has known embryotoxic effects in animals.

Clonopin: *see* CLONAZEPAM

CLOTRIMAZOLE (Lotrimin 1% cream, lotion, or solution, Mycelex 1% cream; *see also* Lotrisone topical cream)

Dose: Massage into skin bid.

Actions: Topical antifungal agent.

COBALAMIN (VITAMIN B₁₂, as either CYANOCOBALAMIN or HYDROXOCOBALAMIN)

Dose: Regimens for replacement therapy vary considerably but are most likely clinically equivalent.

One reasonable regimen is: Either cyanocobalamin or hydroxocobalamin 100–1000 μg IM daily for 7 days, then once or twice per week for 1–2 months or until hematocrit is normal.

Patients with neurologic manifestations should receive 1000 μg for at least the first week.

Patients with pernicious anemia may require chronic treatment at, e.g., 100 μg IM monthly.

Patients with malabsorption may need chronic treatment at, e.g., 1000 μg IM monthly.

Pearls: Symptoms of vitamin B$_{12}$ deficiency include megaloblastic anemia, glossitis, and neurologic dysfunction (paresthesias, ataxia, spastic motor weakness, or reduced mentation).

CODEINE (see also Robitussin A-C, Tylenol with Codeine)

Dose: Use dependent.
Analgesia: 15–60 mg PO, SQ, or IM q4–6h.
Cough suppression: 15–30 mg PO q4–6h.

Preparations: 15, 30, and 60 mg tablets; 30 mg/mL vials for injection.

Actions: Morphine derivative; used to treat pain. Also has antitussive properties and can be used to treat persistent cough.

Clearance: Metabolized via liver (in part to morphine).
Slightly reduce dosage in impaired renal function.
Decrease dosage in liver disease.

Side Effects: Drowsiness, sedation, respiratory depression, nausea and vomiting, constipation.

Pearls: Cost $$–$$$ ($\approx$$30 retail/100 tablets).
Pregnancy category C.

Cogentin: see BENZTROPINE

Colace: see DOCUSATE SODIUM

COLCHICINE

Dose: Use dependent.

Acute gout attack, PO: 1 or 2 tablets initially, then 1 tablet q1h or 2 tablets q2h until pain resolves or diarrhea occurs; max, 6–8 tablets per attack.

Acute gout attack, IV: 2 mg infused slowly (over 2–5 min); may repeat 1–2 mg in 6 h if indicated; max, 4 mg IV.

Prophylaxis: 1 tablet PO bid.

Preparations: 0.5 and 0.6 mg tablets (0.6 mg tablets are usually prescribed); 0.5 mg/mL vials for injection.

Actions: Anti-inflammatory agent that impairs leukocyte chemotaxis and synovial cell phagocytosis; used to treat gout.

Clearance: Renal excreted.

Slightly reduce dosage in ESRD.

No change in dosage needed for liver disease.

Supplemental dose not required after HD.

Side Effects: Nausea and vomiting, abdominal pain, frequent diarrhea. Extravasation can lead to tissue necrosis. Aplastic anemia and agranulocytosis can occur with prolonged use.

Drug Interactions: Decreases absorption of vitamin B_{12}. Phenylbutazone can increase risk of depressed CBC.

Pearls: Cost \$ (PO ≈\$5 retail/100 tablets).

Avoid IV extravasation; some physicians discourage IV administration unless absolutely indicated.

Most effective when used within 24 h of onset of attack.

Colestid: see COLESTIPOL

COLESTIPOL (Colestid)

Dose: 15–30 g PO daily, given in divided doses bid–qid before meals.

Preparations: 5 g packets and 500 g bottles.

Actions: Anion exchange resin, similar to cholestyramine, that binds bile acids; used to treat hypercholesterolemia.

Side Effects: Constipation, GI discomfort.

Drug Interactions: Can reduce absorption of propranolol, chlorthiazide, tetracycline, and digoxin.

Pearls: Cost $$$$ ($\approx$\$3–\$4/d retail); similar in cost to cholestyramine.

Compazine: *see* PROCHLORPERAZINE

Contac (CHLORPHENIRAMINE + PHENYLPROPANOLAMINE)

Dose: 1 caplet or capsule PO q12h prn.

Actions: Combination antihistamine and sympathomimetic.

Cordarone: *see* AMIODARONE

Corgard: *see* NADOLOL

CORTISONE (Cortone Acetate)

Dose: Initial, 25–300 mg PO or IM qd; chronic therapy, 35–70 mg PO qd.

Preparations: 5, 10, and 25 mg tablets; 25 mg/mL vials.

Actions: Synthetic corticosteroid; used primarily to treat adrenocortical insufficiency.

Clearance: Metabolized via liver.
No change in dosage needed for impaired renal function.
Dosage adjustment probably *not* needed in liver disease.
Supplemental dose not required after HD.

Pearls: Cost $$ (≈$0.30/d retail).
Can mask signs of infection.
With chronic use, patients may need "stress-dose" steroids during acute stress (such as infection, etc.).
Pregnancy category not established.

Relative activity of corticosteroids:

	Relative glucocorticoid and anti-inflammatory activity	*Relative mineralocorticoid activity*
cortisone	0.8	0.8
hydrocortisone	1.0	1.0
prednisone	4.0	0.8
triamcinolone	5.0	0.0
methylprednisolone	5.0	0.5
dexamethasone	25–30	0.0

Cortisporin Cream (POLYMYXIN B, NEOMYCIN + HYDROCORTISONE)

Dose: Apply small quantity topically bid–qid.

Preparations: 7.5 g tube.

Actions: Combination topical antibiotic and steroid.

Side Effects: Local irritation, skin sensitization and skin reactions, possible ototoxicity, nephrotoxicity, or adrenocortical suppression.

Pearls: Cost $$ (tube ≈$18 retail).

Cortisporin Ointment (POLYMYXIN B, BACITRACIN, NEOMYCIN + HYDROCORTISONE)

Dose: Apply thin film to skin bid–qid.

Preparations: 0.5 oz tube with applicator tip.

Actions: Combination topical antibiotic and steroid.

Side Effects: Local irritation, skin sensitization and skin reactions, possible ototoxicity, nephrotoxicity, and adrenocortical suppression.

Pearls: Cost $$$ (tube ≈$30 retail).
  Pregnancy category C.

Cortisporin Ophthalmic Ointment (POLYMYXIN B, BACITRACIN, NEOMYCIN + HYDROCORTISONE)

Dose: 1 or 2 drops (written "gtt") into the eye q3–4h.

Preparations: 1/8 oz tube.

Actions: Combination antibiotic; used to treat superficial ocular infections and inflammatory ocular conditions.

Pearls: Cost $$ (tube: generic ≈$10 retail, Cortisporin ≈$20 retail).
  Pregnancy category C.

Cortisporin Ophthalmic Suspension (HYDROCORTISONE, NEOMYCIN + POLYMYXIN B)

Dose: Insert 1/2 inch into the conjunctival sac tid–qid.

Preparations: 7.5 mL dispenser bottle.

Actions: Combination antibiotic and anti-inflammatory agent; used to treat inflammatory ocular conditions and infections.

Cortisporin Otic Solution (POLYMYXIN B, NEOMYCIN + HYDROCORTISONE)

Dose: 4 drops (written "gtt") into the ear tid–qid.

Preparations: 10 mL bottle with dropper.

Actions: Topical antibiotic and steroid; used to treat infections of the external auditory canal.

Pearls: Cost: generic $, Cortisporin $$$ (bottle: generic ≈$6 retail; Cortisporin ≈$24 retail).

Cortone Acetate: *see* **CORTISONE**

Coumadin: *see* **WARFARIN**

CROMOLYN SODIUM (Intal, Nasalcrom, Opticrom)

Dose: Route dependent.
Aerosol: Inhale 2 puffs qid.
Powder: Inhale 20 mg (in a capsule) qid.
Spray: Spray into each nostril 2–6 times daily.

Preparations: 8.1 and 14.2 g aerosol canisters; 20 mg capsules; 20 mg/2 mL ampules of nebulizer solution.

Actions: Medication with antiasthmatic and antiallergic properties, possibly related to mast cell stabilization; used in chronic (not acute) treatment of certain types of asthma and allergic conditions.

Pearls: Cost $$$$ (14.2 g inhaler ≈$55 retail); no generic form available.
Can take 2–4 weeks to achieve maximal effect.
Pregnancy category B.

CYANOCOBALAMIN: *see* COBALAMIN

CYCLOBENZAPRINE (Flexeril)

Dose: 5–20 mg PO tid; usually effective at 10 mg PO tid.

Preparations: 10 mg tablets.

Actions: Tricyclic amine; used to treat skeletal muscle spasm of local origin.

Clearance: Metabolized via liver; renal excreted.

Side Effects: Drowsiness, dizziness, dry mouth and other anticholinergic effects. Can have tricyclic-like proarrhythmic effects.

Cautions: Contraindicated in patients who have taken MAOI within 14 days and in patients with hyperthyroidism, recent MI, significant heart block, conduction disturbances, or arrhythmias.

Pearls: Cost $$$ (100 tablets retail: generic ≈$55, Flexeril ≈$85).

Warn patients of possible sedative effects. Consider beginning patients on 5 mg (half of the 10 mg tablet) PO TID.

Pregnancy category B.

Cyclogyl: see CYCLOPENTOLATE

CYCLOPENTOLATE (Cyclogyl)

Dose: Instill 1 drop (written "gtt") in the eye; may be used up to qid for iritis.

Preparations: 2, 5, and 15 mL containers; available in 0.5, 1.0, and 2.0% solutions.

Actions: Cycloplegic agent that paralyzes sphincter and ciliary muscle, dilating the pupil and inhibiting painful ciliary muscle spasm; used to treat iritis.

Side Effects (local): Increased intraocular pressure.

Side Effects (systemic): Hallucinations, psychotic reactions, other CNS disturbances.

Cautions: Use with caution in patients who may have increased intraocular pressure or narrow-angle glaucoma.

Pearls: Caution patients not to drive or engage in other hazardous activities while pupils are dilated (paralysis of ciliary muscle causes inability to focus the eyes).

Onset of action 30 min; duration of action up to 12–24 h.

Pregnancy category not established.

CYCLOPHOSPHAMIDE (Cytoxan)

Dose: Extremely variable; tumor dependent. May be given PO or IV (not qhs).

Preparations: 25 and 50 mg tablets; multiple IV preparations.

Actions: Antineoplastic alkylating agent that crosslinks tumor cell DNA; used to treat malignancies.

Clearance: Activated and metabolized via liver; 5–25% excreted unchanged in urine.

PDR notes no increase in toxicity in renal failure; other sources recommend slightly reducing dosage or increasing dosing interval, or decreasing dose when CrCl <10 mL/min.

Liver failure may affect both its activation to the active form and its metabolism to inactive products.

Supplemental dose suggested after HD.

Side Effects: Hemorrhagic cystitis and ureteritis, fibrosis of urinary bladder and renal tubules, immune suppression, alopecia, nausea and vomiting, anorexia, abdominal discomfort, diarrhea, myelosuppression, impaired wound healing, sterility, rare anaphylactoid reaction, pulmonary fibrosis (with prolonged high-dose therapy), SIADH, cardiomyopathy, rare hemorrhagic colitis, ulcer of oral mucosa, jaundice.

Drug Interactions: Potentiates doxorubicin-induced cardiotoxicity. Its anticholinergic effects potentiate the effect of succinylcholine. Phenobarbital increases its leukopenic effects.

Caution: Is known to harm the fetus when taken during pregnancy.

Pearls: Cost $$$ (50 mg PO ≈$225 wholesale/100 tablets, 500 mg IV ≈$20 wholesale).

Nadir occurs and WBC recovery usually begins 7–10 days after cessation of therapy.

May necessitate additional steroids in adrenalectomized patients.

Secondary cancers are associated with its use.

Encourage generous fluid intake (2–3 quarts daily) and frequent voiding following treatment (to reduce risk of hemorrhagic cystitis).

The cytoprotective agent mesna may be used to prevent hemorrhagic cystitis.

Pregnancy category D.

CYCLOSPORINE (CYCLOSPORIN A)

Dose: Variable initially; maintenance, 5–10 mg/kg PO qd.

Preparations: 25 mg capsules; 50 mL bottles containing 100 mg/mL oral suspension; 5 mL ampules containing 50 mg/mL.

Actions: Immunosuppressant that prolongs survival of allogenic organ transplants, most likely through T cell suppression; used to treat transplant recipients.

Clearance: Extensively metabolized and excreted in bile; only 6% excreted in urine.
  No change in dosage needed for impaired renal function.
  May need to reduce dosage in liver disease.
  Supplemental dose not required after HD or PD.

Side Effects: Impaired renal function and nephrotoxicity, hepatotoxicity, hyperkalemia, tremor, hirsuitism, hypertension, hyperplasia of gums.

Drug Interactions: Can significantly increase K^+ when used with K^+-sparing diuretics. Somatostatin, phenytoin, phenobarbital, rifampin, and IV trimethoprim reduce its serum level. Danazol, diltiazem, ketoconazole, methylprednisolone, metoclopramide, and prednisolone raise its serum level.

Pearls: Cost $$$$ (PO ≈$20/d wholesale).
  Follow LFTs and renal function; periodically check cyclosporine levels.
  Adjunct steroid therapy is usually needed.
  Pregnancy category C.

CYPROHEPTADINE (Periactin)

Dose: Usual, 4 mg PO tid–qid; range, 4–32 mg PO daily.

Preparations: 4 mg scored tablets; 473 mL bottles containing 2 mg/5 mL (1 tsp).

Actions: Antihistamine with anticholinergic, sedative, and serotonin-antagonistic effects; used to treat allergic disorders.

Clearance: Renal metabolized and excreted; elimination is decreased in renal insufficiency.
  Probably need to adjust dosage in impaired renal function.

Side Effects: Drowsiness, dry mouth, urinary symptoms, dizziness, irritability, blurred vision or diplopia, tachycardia or palpitations, hypotension, many other CNS effects.

Drug Interactions: MAOI prolong and intensify its anti-cholinergic effects. Potentiates CNS depressant effects of other CNS depressants. Effects may be modified when used with other serotoninergic drugs.

Cautions: Contraindicated in patients with increased intraocular pressure, symptomatic benign prostatic hypertrophy, bladder neck obstruction, or upper GI stenoses, in elderly or debilitated patients, and in patients taking MAOI.

Use with caution in patients with cardiovascular disease, hypertension, history of bronchial asthma, or hyperthyroidism.

Pearls: Cost: generic $$, Periactin $$$ (generic $\approx$$0.30/d retail, Periactin $\approx$$1.20/d retail).

Caution patients about its sedative effects and warn them to avoid activities requiring mental alertness and coordination, such as driving a car or operating heavy machinery.

Pregnancy category B.

CYTARABINE: see CYTOSINE ARABINOSIDE
Cytosar-U: see CYTOSINE ARABINOSIDE

CYTOSINE ARABINOSIDE (ARA-C, CYTARABINE, Cytosar-U)

Dose: Tumor dependent; often 100 mg/m^2/d by continuous infusion for 7 days.

Actions: Antineoplastic agent that is cytotoxic to cells undergoing DNA synthesis (S-phase); used to treat malignancies.

Clearance: Metabolized via liver to inactive ara-U.

No change in dosage needed for impaired renal function.

One source recommends reducing dosage in liver disease; a second recommends only following the patient carefully.

Side Effects: Bone marrow suppression, nausea and vomiting, anorexia, fever, rash, oral and anal inflammation or ulceration, thrombophlebitis, elevated LFTs, hyperuricemia, "cytarabine syndrome" (flu-like syndrome with fever, myalgia, arthralgia, bone pain, chest pain, rash, conjunctivitis, and malaise).

Drug Interactions: Can alter excretion of digoxin. Can interfere with gentamicin therapy for *K. pneumoniae.*

Cautions: Should not be used in pregnant or potentially pregnant patients.

Pearls: Cost $$ (100 mg ≈$6 retail).
May be given intrathecally.
A biphasic decrease in WBCs will occur: initial decline is seen within 24 h with nadir at days 7–9 followed by a second, deeper depression with nadir at days 15–24, then rapid rise to above baseline in next 10 days.
Periodically check CBC, LFTs, renal function, and uric acid levels.
"Cytarabine syndrome" occurs 6–12 h after administration and can be treated with steroids.
Is known to harm the fetus when taken during pregnancy.

Cytotec: see MISOPROSTOL

Cytoxan: see CYCLOPHOSPHAMIDE

Dalmane: see FLURAZEPAM

Dantrium: see DANTROLENE

DANTROLENE (Dantrium)

Dose: Initial, 25 mg PO qd; max, 100 mg PO bid–qid.

Preparations: 25, 50, and 100 mg capsules.

Actions: Muscle relaxant; used to treat spasticity.

Side Effects: Hepatotoxicity.

Pearls: Cost $$$$ (≈$2.50/d retail).

DAPSONE

Dose: Disease dependent.
PCP: 100 mg PO qd; one source recommends giving trimethoprim 5 mg/kg PO qid with dapsone for PCP therapy.

Preparations: 25 and 100 mg.

Actions: Antibiotic that may act by inhibiting folate synthesis; used to treat various infections.

Clearance: Acetylated in liver; undergoes enterohepatic circulation; excreted in urine.

Side Effects: Dose-related hemolysis, agranulocytosis, aplastic anemia, elevated LFTs, peripheral neuropathy.

Drug Interactions: Rifampin markedly increases its clearance and reduces its serum level. Folic acid antagonists may increase chance of hematologic reactions. Probenecid reduces its renal excretion, so dosage should be adjusted.

Cautions: Use with caution in G6PD deficiency and sulfone hypersensitivity.

Pearls: Cost $$$ ($\approx$$1/tablet retail).
Warn patients to report any signs of infection.
Follow CBC weekly for the first month, then monthly for 6 months, then semiannually.
Follow LFTs.
Pregnancy category C.

Darvocet N-50, Darvocet N-100 (PROPOXYPHENE + ACETAMINOPHEN)

Dose: 2 tablets of Darvocet-N 50 or 1 tablet of Darvocet-N 100 q4h PO prn.

Preparations: Each Darvocet-N 50 tablet contains 50 mg propoxyphene and 325 mg acetaminophen; each Darvocet-N 100 contains 100 mg propoxyphene and 650 mg acetaminophen.

Actions: Weak narcotic analgesic with antipyretic actions; used to treat mild pain.

Clearance: Metabolized primarily via liver.
Avoid in ESRD (metabolites that have lidocaine-like effects will accumulate).
Reduce dosage in liver disease.

Cautions: Use with caution in liver disease (acetaminophen may be hepatotoxic in high doses).

Pearls: Cost $$$ (100 tablets retail: 50 mg generic ≈$20, 50 mg Darvocet N-50 ≈$33, 100 mg generic ≈$20, 100 mg Darvocet N-100 ≈$50).
Pregnancy category not established.

Darvon, Darvon-N: see PROPOXYPHENE

DAUNORUBICIN (Cerubidine)

Dose: Disease dependent. Often given 25–45 mg/m²/d IV for 3 days, then the same dose given for 2 days on subsequent courses; lower doses may be given in elderly patients.

Preparations: 20 mg vials also containing 100 mg mannitol.

Actions: Cytotoxic anthracycline that impairs DNA synthesis by inserting itself between DNA base pairs; used to treat many neoplastic diseases.

Clearance: 20–30% of dose is excreted in bile; metabolized to the active metabolite daunorubicinol.
Reduce dosage in liver or kidney disease based on bilirubin and creatinine levels, as described in *PDR*.

Side Effects: Cardiotoxicity, myelosuppression, frequent nausea and vomiting, frequent stomatitis, alopecia, severe local skin necrosis when extravasated, hyperuricemia when treating leukemia.

Pearls: Cost $$$ (20 mg ≈$117).
Myelosuppression and cardiotoxicity are dose-limiting side effects.
WBC and platelet nadirs usually occur 9–14 days after treatment with nearly complete recovery by 3 weeks.
The major cardiotoxicity is CHF; patients with preexisting heart disease or previously treated with daunorubicin are at increased risk.
Cardiotoxicity is rare with cumulative doses <550 mg/m².
Signs suggestive of cardiotoxicity are reduced ejection fraction or >30% decrease in QRS voltage in limb leads.
Obtain ejection fraction and ECG prior to each treatment.
Warn patients that it colors urine red up to 2 days after administration.
Pregnancy category D.

DDAVP: *see* **DESMOPRESSIN**

Decadron: *see* **DEXAMETHASONE**

Delsym (DEXTROMETHORPHAN)

Dose: Age dependent.
    Adults and children >12 years: 2 tsp PO q12h.
    Children 6–11 years: 1 tsp PO q12h.
    Children 2–5 years: 1/2 tsp PO q12h.

Preparations: 3 oz bottles containing 30 mg/5 mL (1 tsp) dextromethorphan.

Actions: Centrally acting non-narcotic cough suppressant.

Drug Interactions: Concomitant use with MAOI can cause hyperpyretic crisis.

Delta-Cortef: *see* **PREDNISOLONE**

Demerol: *see* **MEPERIDINE**

Deodorized Tincture of Opium (DTO)

Dose: 0.5–1.5 mL PO or via NG or feeding tube tid–qid.

Preparations: Tincture containing 10% opium and 19% ethanol.

Actions: Non-narcotic opioid; used to treat diarrhea.

Pearls: Do not confuse with Paregoric (camphorated tincture of opium).

Depakene: *see* **VALPROIC ACID**

Depakote: *see* **VALPROIC ACID**

Depo-Medrol: *see* **METHYLPREDNISOLONE**

DESIPRAMINE (Norpramin)

Dose: Usual, 100–200 mg PO qd (25–100 mg PO qd in elderly patients); max, 300 mg PO qd.

Preparations: 25 and 50 mg capsules; 10, 25, 50, 75, 100, and 150 mg tablets.

Actions: Tricyclic antidepressant that may work by blocking reuptake of neurotransmitters, especially norepinephrine; used to treat depression.

Clearance: Metabolized predominantly via liver; usually metabolized more slowly in elderly patients.
No change in dosage needed for impaired renal function.
Supplemental dose not required after HD or PD.

Side Effects: Numerous hemodynamic, conduction, psychiatric, neurologic, and anticholinergic effects.

Drug Interactions: Decreases antihypertensive effect of clonidine, methyldopa, and guanethidine. Cimetidine, phenothiazines, and psychostimulants raise its serum level. Discontinuing cimetidine may reduce its serum level. Cigarette smoking as well as alcohol, barbiturates, and several other substances induce hepatic enzyme activity and depress its serum level. Coadministration with MAOI may lead to hypertensive crisis, convulsions, and death.

Cautions: Contraindicated within 2 weeks of MAOI therapy and in acute post-MI recovery period.
Use with caution in patients with cardiovascular disease, thyroid disease, or history of urine retention, glaucoma, or seizures (lowers the seizure threshold).

Pearls: Cost: generic $$$, Norpramin $$$$ (100 tablets retail: 100 mg generic ≈$60, 100 mg Norpramin ≈$160).
Earliest therapeutic effect may be seen in 2–5 days; full benefit usually is obtained after 2–3 weeks.
Follow ECG (especially with higher doses) for prolongation of QRS or QT interval, which best correlate with impending toxicity.
Signs and symptoms of overdose include agitation, stupor, coma, hypotension, shock, renal shutdown, seizures, hyperactive reflexes, muscle rigidity, hyperpyrexia, vomiting, respiratory depression, and impaired conduction and arrhythmias on ECG.
Pregnancy category not established.

DESMOPRESSIN (DDAVP)

Dose: Bleeding disorders: 0.3 μg/kg diluted in 50 mL NS, injected slowly IV over 15–30 min.

Preparations: 4.0 μg/mL ampules for injection.

Actions: Synthetic analog of arginine vasopressin; used to treat certain types of platelet dysfunction. Mechanism of action may be related to increasing factor VIII levels in plasma.

Side Effects: Infrequent headaches, nausea or GI distress, local burning and erythema, facial flushing, BP changes. Watch for possible water intoxication or hyponatremia.

Pearls: Monitor BP during injection.
Pregnancy category B.

Desyrel: see TRAZODONE

DEXAMETHASONE (Decadron)

Dose: Disease or use dependent.
Cerebral edema: 10 mg IM or IV initially, then 6 mg IM or IV q6h (a somewhat arbitrary dose that is frequently recommended); may also give 0.75–9.0 mg PO qd.

Dexamethasone suppression test for outpatient screening: Give 1 mg PO at 11:00 PM and draw plasma cortisol level at 8:00 AM the next day.

Dexamethasone suppression test for inpatient workup of Cushing's syndrome: Establish baseline by giving no drug on days 1 and 2. On days 3 and 4 give 0.5 mg PO q6h (low dose), and on days 5 and 6 give 2.0 mg PO q6h (high dose). Measure consecutive 24hour urinary free cortisol levels on each of the 6 days.

Preparations: 0.25, 0.5, 0.75, 1.5, 4.0, and 6.0 mg tablets; 4 and 24 mg/mL vials for injection.

Actions: Corticosteroid with potent anti-inflammatory actions; used primarily to treat inflammatory or allergic conditions.

Clearance: Metabolized via liver.
No change in dosage needed for impaired renal function, and probably not for liver disease.

Side Effects: Increased glucose intolerance, psychiatric derangements ("steroid psychosis"), increased catabolism, worsening azotemia.

Drug Interactions: Reduces hypoglycemic actions of insulin and oral hypoglycemic agents. Can increase or decrease PT in patients taking warfarin. Phenytoin, phenobarbital, and rifampin increase its clearance and reduce its serum level.

Pearls: Cost $$ (IV ≈$20/d retail).
Can mask signs of infection.
Patients may need "stress doses" in times of stress.
Used more frequently in cerebral edema caused by tumor; used less commonly, if at all, for edema secondary to cerebral hemorrhage or anoxic encephalopathy.
Pregnancy category not established.

Relative steroid activity:

	Relative anti-inflammatory and glucocorticoid activity	Relative mineralocorticoid activity
dexamethasone	25–30	0.0
hydrocortisone	1.0	1.0
prednisone	4.0	0.8
methylprednisolone	5.0	0.5

DEXTROMETHORPHAN: see Delsym, Robitussin-CF, Robitussin-DM

DiaBeta: see GLYBURIDE

Diabinese: see CHLORPROPAMIDE

Diamox: see ACETAZOLAMIDE

DIAZEPAM (Valium)

Dose: Disease dependent.
  Acute seizure: 5–10 mg IV initially (2.5 mg IV is sometimes given as starting dose in frail or elderly patients); may repeat q10–15min to maximum of 30 mg. Inject gradually (no faster than 5 mg/min).
  Muscle spasm: 5–10 mg IM or IV.
  Alcohol withdrawal: 5–10 mg IM or IV initially; regimens from different sources vary markedly after this, with most suggesting repeat doses of 5–10 mg IM or IV at intervals varying from q5–10min to q3–4h depending on severity of withdrawal symptoms.
  Acute anxiety: 2–10 mg IM or IV.
  Chronic anxiety: 2–10 mg PO bid–qid.

Preparations: 2, 5, and 10 mg tablets; 15 mg sustained-release tablets; 5 mg/5 mL (1 tsp) and 5 mg/mL solutions; 5 mg/mL for injection.

Actions: Benzodiazepine with anxiolytic, antiseizure, and anti-spasmodic action; used to treat anxiety, seizures, and muscle spasms.

Clearance: Metabolized via liver.
  Active metabolite is renal excreted, but no change in dosage is suggested for renal disease.
  Reduce dosage or increase dosing interval in liver disease.
  Supplemental dose not required after HD.

Side Effects: Drowsiness, fatigue, ataxia, local thrombosis and phlebitis.

Drug Interactions: Cimetidine reduces its clearance. Potentiates CNS depressant effects of other CNS depressants.

Cautions: Contraindicated in untreated patients with narrow- or open-angle glaucoma.
  Use with caution in elderly patients.
  Generally should not be used in pregnant or potentially pregnant patients.

Pearls: Cost: generic $, Valium $$$ (100 tablets retail: 5 mg PO generic ≈$13, 5 mg PO Valium ≈$50).

Abrupt discontinuance can cause withdrawal reactions.

Antiseizure effects when used IV may be short-lived; consider starting a longer-acting anticonvulsant.

Signs and symptoms of overdose include somnolence, confusion, coma, and diminished reflexes.

Almost always avoid in pregnant or potentially pregnant patients.

DICLOXACILLIN

Dose: 0.5–1.0 g PO qid.

Preparations: 250 and 500 mg capsules; 62.5 mg/5 mL (1 tsp) solution bottles to make 100 mL.

Actions: Bactericidal β-lactamase–resistant penicillin that inhibits cell wall synthesis. Good gram (+) coverage including staph and strep (but *not* MRSA or enterococci); *no* gram (−) coverage; poor anaerobic coverage.

Clearance: Metabolized via liver; renal excreted.

No change in dosage needed for impaired renal function or liver disease.

Supplemental dose not required after HD.

Side Effects: GI discomfort, rash, elevated LFTs, cholestatic jaundice.

Cautions: Contraindicated in patients with penicillin allergy.

Pearls: Cost $$ (≈$20/wk retail); see under Penicillin for a comparison of weekly costs for brand-name and generic oral antibiotics.

Pregnancy category B.

Diflucan: see FLUCONAZOLE

DIFLUNISAL (Dolobid)

Dose: Treatment dependent.
  Arthritis: 250–500 mg PO bid.
  Mild to moderate pain: 1000 mg PO initially, then 500 mg PO bid–tid.

Preparations: 250 and 500 mg tablets.

Actions: Nonsteroidal anti-inflammatory agent; used to treat mild to moderate pain and inflammatory conditions.

Side Effects: GI distress and upper GI bleeding, rash, headache, interstitial nephritis and renal papillary necrosis, hypersensitivity reactions.

Drug Interactions: Raises serum level of acetaminophen by 50%. Lowers excretion of methotrexate and increases its toxicity. Increases toxicity of cyclosporine. Chronic coadministration with antacids may reduce its serum level. Prolongs PT in some patients taking warfarin.

Cautions: Contraindicated in patients with history of hypersensitivity to aspirin or other NSAID.
  Use with caution, if at all, in patients with history of upper GI bleeding.

Pearls: Cost $$$$ (≈$2/d retail).
  500 mg diflunisal has analgesic effect similar to that of 650 mg of ASA or acetaminophen.
  Has little antipyretic activity.
  Pregnancy category C.

DIGOXIN (Lanoxin)

Dose: Situation dependent.
  In-patient management of atrial fibrillation or congestive heart failure: Usual regimen is 0.25–0.50 mg IV initially, followed by further doses of 0.25 mg IV q6–8h until rate control is achieved or total of 1.0 mg has been given.
  Out-patient management of congestive heart failure: Loading dose of 1.0–1.5 mg PO, given in divided doses over 1–3 days; maintenance, usually 0.125–0.25 mg PO or IV qod–qd depending on renal function and clinical response.

Preparations: 0.125, 0.25, and 0.5 mg tablets; 0.05, 0.1, and 0.2 mg capsules; 0.05 mg/mL elixir; 0.1 and 0.25 mg/mL for injection.

Actions: Cardiac glycoside with direct inotropic and indirect vagomimetic effects; used to treat CHF and for rate control of supraventricular arrhythmias involving the AV node (atrial fibrillation or flutter, SVT).

Clearance: Renal excreted.

Moderately to markedly reduce dosage or moderately increase dosing interval in impaired renal function; some sources recommend decreasing *loading* dose by 50% in ESRD.

No change in dosage needed for liver disease.

Supplemental dose not required after HD or PD.

Side Effects: Ventricular tachycardia or fibrillation, paroxysmal atrial tachycardia with block, sinoatrial and AV block, fatigue, dizziness, anorexia, nausea and vomiting, gynecomastia.

Drug Interactions: Quinidine, verapamil, diltiazem, amiodarone, disopyramide, propafenone, flecainide, erythromycin, tetracycline, and phenytoin all raise its serum level. Antacids, kaopectate, cholestyramine, and sucralfate reduce its intestinal absorption.

Cautions: Use with caution in patients with sick sinus syndrome, WPW, or IHSS.

Pearls: Cost $ ($\approx$$7 retail/100 tablets); generic and brand names same price.

Check K^+ level before use.

Cardioversion is contraindicated in digoxin toxicity.

Can cause nonischemic-mediated ECG changes during exercise testing and thus lead to false (+) test results.

Although HD generally does not remove significant amounts of digoxin, it may be useful in overdose (especially if K^+ is substantially elevated).

At higher doses, digoxin increases sympathetic outflow from the CNS, which may contribute to digitalis cardiotoxicity.

Usual therapeutic level for (+) inotropy is 0.8–2.0 ng/mL.

IV digoxin will take several hours to slow the ventricullar response in atrial fibrillation. Thus if acute rate control is required, consider using the IV preparations of verapamil, diltiazem, esmolol, propanol, atenol, or metoprolol.

Pregnancy category C.

DIHYDROXYALUMINUM SODIUM CARBONATE: see Rolaids

Dilantin: see PHENYTOIN

Dilaudid: see HYDROMORPHNE

DILTIAZEM [IV] (Cardizem; see also DILTIAZEM [PO])

Dose: Initial, 0.25 mg/kg (actual body weight) over 2 min; if response is inadequate, wait 15 min from first injection and then give 0.35 mg/kg (actual body weight) over 2 min.
Maintenance: Begin constant infusion of 5–15 mg/h.

Actions: Injectable calcium-channel blocker; used to convert paroxysmal SVT to sinus rhythm and to control ventricular rate during atrial fibrillation or flutter.

Clearance: Metabolized primarily via liver.
Manufacturer suggests using with caution in liver or kidney disease.

Side Effects: Hypotension, vasodilatation and flushing, irritation at injection site, AV block.

Drug Interactions: Can increase bioavailability of propranolol. Theoretically, can have additive effects with digoxin in slowing HR and increasing AV block (although manufacturer reports that this combination of drugs has been well tolerated).

Cautions: Contraindicated in sick sinus syndrome and second- or third-degree AV block except when a functioning ventricular pacemaker is in place.
Contraindicated in patients with severe hypotension, cardiogenic shock, VT, atrial fibrillation or flutter, or an accessory bypass tract such as in WPW syndrome or short PR syndrome.
Be *sure* any wide complex tachycardia is *not* VT before prescribing.
Use with caution in patients with impaired ventricular function.

Pearls: Ventricular rate reduction during atrial fibrillation or flutter usually occurs within 3 min and is maximal within 2–7 min.
Duration of action for the initial bolus is usually 1–3 h.
Patients should undergo continuous ECG monitoring and have frequent BP checks during therapy.
Pregnancy category C.

DILTIAZEM [PO] (Cardizem; *see also* DILTIAZEM [IV])

Dose: Preparation dependent.
  Regular pills: 30–90 mg PO tid–qid.
  Cardizem SR: 60–180 mg PO bid.
  Cardizem CD: 180–300 mg PO qd.

Preparations: 30, 60, 90, and 120 mg regular tablets; 60, 90, 120, and 180 mg long-acting Cardizem SR tablets; 180, 240, and 300 mg once-a-day Cardizem CD capsules.

Actions: Calcium-channel blocker; used to treat angina and hypertension.

Clearance: Metabolized via liver.
  No change in dosage needed for impaired renal function.

Side Effects: Sinoatrial and AV block, headache, vasodilatation-induced peripheral edema, flushing, CHF, bradycardia.

Cautions: Use with caution in patients with depressed LV ejection fraction or AV block.

Drug Interactions: Can raise serum level of digoxin. Can increase bioavailability of propranolol. Cimetidine raises its serum level. Concomitant use with β-blockers or digoxin increases risk of AV block.

Cautions: Use with caution in patients with depressed LV ejection fraction or AV block.

Pearls: Cost $$$ ($1.00–$1.80/d retail).
  Pregnancy category C.

DIMENHYDRINATE (Dramamine)

Dose: Route dependent.
  PO: 50–100 mg q4–6h; max, 400 mg daily.
  Liquid (12.5 mg/5 mL): 4–8 tsp q4–6h prn, not to exceed 32 tsp in 24 h; (15.62 mg/5 mL): 4–7 tsp q4–6h prn, not to exceed 26 tsp in 24 h.
  IM or IV: 50 mg prn.

Preparations: 50 mg tablets, capsules, and chewable tablets; 12.5 and 15.62 mg/5 mL (1 tsp) liquid; 50 mg/mL injection.

Actions: Diphenhydramine derivative; used to treat motion sickness.

Side Effects: Drowsiness, anticholinergic side effects.

Pearls: Cost: generic $, Dramamine $$$ (12 tablets retail: 50 mg generic ≈$2, 50 mg Dramamine ≈$8).
First PO dose should be taken 30 min to 1 h prior to trip.
Sold over-the-counter without a prescription.
Pregnancy category B.

Dipentum: see OLSALAZINE SODIUM

DIPHENHYDRAMINE (Benadryl)

Dose: Disease or use dependent.
Antihistamine: 25–50 mg PO tid–qid.
Prophylaxis for motion sickness: 50 mg PO 30 min before exposure.
Sleep aid: 25–50 mg PO qhs.
Anaphylaxis or parkinsonism: 10–50 mg deep IM or IV.

Preparations: 25 and 50 mg tablets; 12.5 mg/5 mL (1 tsp) elixir; 12.5 mg/5 mL (1 tsp) syrup; 10 and 50 mg/mL injection.

Actions: Antihistamine with anticholinergic and sedative properties; used to treat allergic conditions, motion sickness, and cough, as a hypnotic, and as an antiparkinsonian agent (for both idiopathic and drug-induced disease).

Clearance: Metabolized via liver.
Slightly increase dosing interval in impaired renal function.
Reduce dosage in liver disease.

Side Effects: Drowsiness and sedation, epigastric distress, thickening of bronchial secretions, dry mouth, urine retention, psychotic reactions.

Drug Interactions: Severe adverse reactions when used with MAOI.

Cautions: Contraindicated in patients taking MAOI. Use with caution in narrow-angle glaucoma, symptomatic prostate hypertrophy, or bladder neck obstruction.

Use with caution (because of atropine-like effect) in patients with history of bronchial asthma, elevated intraocular pressure, hyperthyroidism, hypertension, or cardiovascular disease.

Pearls: Cost $ (25 mg Benadryl ≈$12 retail/100 tablets).
Sold over-the-counter.
Pregnancy category B.

DIPHENOXYLATE: see Lomotil

DIPIVEFRIN (Propine ophthalmic solution)

Dose: 1 drop (written "gtt") of 0.1% solution in the eye q12h.

Preparations: 5, 10, and 15 mL of 0.1% solution.

Actions: Ophthalmic pro-drug that is converted to epinephrine, which then lowers intraocular pressure by increasing outflow of aqueous humor and reducing its production; used to treat open-angle glaucoma.

Side Effects (local): Injections, burning, stinging.

Side Effects (systemic): Tachycardia, arrhythmias, hypertension.

Pearls: To decrease systemic absorption, compress the lacrimal sac with a finger after instilling drops.
Pregnancy category B.

DIPYRIDAMOLE (Persantine)

Dose: 75–100 mg PO tid.

Preparations: 25, 50, and 75 mg tablets.

Actions: Medication that inhibits platelet aggregation and increases coronary blood flow; usually used in patients following coronary bypass surgery.

Clearance: Metabolized via liver.
No change in dosage needed for impaired renal function.

Side Effects: Rare hypotension, dizziness, abdominal pain, GI upset, rash.

Pearls: Cost: generic $$, Persantine $$$$ (generic ≈$0.36/d retail, Persantine ≈$1.70/d retail).

Does not increase risk of bleeding when given to patients taking warfarin.

Pregnancy category B.

Disalcid: see SALSALATE

DISOPYRAMIDE (Norpace)

Dose: Delivery dependent.
Regular pills: 100–200 mg q6–8h.
Long-acting pills: 100–300 mg PO bid of Norpace CR.

Preparations: 100 and 150 mg regular tablets; 100 and 150 mg long-acting tablets.

Actions: Type Ia antiarrhythmic; used to treat ventricular and supraventricular arrhythmias.

Clearance: Some liver metabolism; primarily renal excreted.
Moderately increase dosing interval in impaired renal function.
May need to adjust dosage in liver dysfunction (because of prolonged $t_{1/2}$).
Supplemental dose suggested after HD.

Side Effects: Substantially reduced ejection fraction, anticholinergic effects, rare hypoglycemia, conduction abnormalities, increased arrhythmias, nausea and vomiting, constipation.

Drug Interactions: Hepatic enzyme inducers decrease its serum level.

Cautions: Use with caution in patients taking β-blockers or calcium-channel blockers.

Pearls: Cost $$$ (generic ≈$1/d retail; Norpace ≈$2/d retail).
Follow corrected QT interval (>25% increase predisposes to development of the ventricular arrhythmia torsades de pointes).

Give an AV blocker prior to use in patients with atrial flutter (not fibrillation).

Usual therapeutic level is 2–5 µg/mL.

Pregnancy category C.

DISULFIRAM (Antabuse)

Dose: 500 mg PO qd for 1–2 weeks, then 250 mg PO qd.

Preparations: 250 and 500 mg scored tablets.

Actions: Antioxidant that blocks oxidation of alcohol, increasing the concentration of acetaldehyde and resulting in an unpleasant reaction; used in aversion therapy for chronic alcoholism.

Drug Interactions: Inhibits metabolism of alcohol, phenytoin, and warfarin.

Cautions: Contraindicated in patients with severe cardiac disease, psychoses, or hypersensitivity to thiuram derivatives.

Contraindicated in patients currently taking metronidazole, chlorpropamide, isoniazid, phenytoin, paraldehyde, alcohol, or alcohol-containing products.

Disulfiram should *never* be administered without a patient's full knowledge and consent.

Pearls: Cost $$ (500 mg Antabuse ≈$75 retail/100 tablets).

When mixed with alcohol, causes flushing, head and neck throbbing, headache, nausea and vomiting, respiratory difficulty, sweating, chest pain, CNS effects, etc.

Patients should carry identification stating that they are receiving disulfiram.

20% of the drug remains 1 week after therapy is discontinued.

Pregnancy category not established.

Ditropan: see OXYBUTYNIN

Diuril: see CHLOROTHIAZIDE

DIVALPROEX SODIUM: see VALPROIC ACID

DOBUTAMINE (Dobutrex)

Dose: Initial, 1–2 μg/kg/min IV; usual, 2.5–10 μg/kg/min IV.

Preparations: 250 mg/20 mL injection.

Actions: β_1-Stimulant that increases inotropy, HR, and BP; used to treat CHF caused by poor systolic function.

Clearance: Metabolized via liver and other tissues.

Side Effects: Elevated BP, substantially increased HR, palpitations, increased arrhythmias, angina, headache, nausea.

Cautions: Contraindicated in IHSS.

Pearls: Cost $$$ (≈$50/d wholesale).
Increases AV conduction and can raise ventricular rate in atrial fibrillation.
May increase insulin requirements.

Dobutrex: see DOBUTAMINE

DOCUSATE SODIUM (Colace; see also Peri-Colace)

Dose: 50–100 mg PO qd–bid.

Preparations: 50 and 100 mg capsules.

Actions: Stool softener (not a laxative).

Side Effects: Minimal.

Pearls: Cost $$ (generic ≈$0.25/d retail, Colace ≈$0.60/d retail).

Dolobid: see DIFLUNISAL

DOPAMINE (Intropin)

Dose: 2.5–20 μg/kg/min.

Preparations: 40, 80, and 160 mg/mL injection.

Actions: Dose dependent. Predominant effect at "renal doses" of 2–4 μg/kg/min is a dopaminergic receptor mediated increase in renal blood flow; at doses of 5–10 μg/kg/min, a β-adrenergic receptor mediated increase in cardiac inotropy; at doses >10 μg/kg/min, an α-adrenergic receptor mediated increase in systemic vascular resistance.

Clearance: Metabolized in liver.

Side Effects: Angina, substantially increased HR, increased PVCs, substantially reduced BP, headache, nausea and vomiting.

Cautions: Use with caution in occlusive vascular disease.

Pearls: Cost $ (≈$6/d wholesale).
Psychotropic drugs can block dopa receptors and reduce its effectiveness.
Doses greater than 10 μg/kg/min can decrease renal perfusion.
Pregnancy category C.

Doral: see QUAZEPAM

DOXAZOSIN (Cardura)

Dose: Initial, 1 mg PO qd; may titrate *stepwise* to 2, 4, 8, or 16 mg PO qd.

Preparations: 1, 2, 4, 8, and 16 mg scored tablets.

Actions: α_1-Receptor blocker that causes peripheral dilation; used to treat hypertension.

Clearance: Extensively metabolized.

Side Effects: Orthostatic hypotension, syncope, vertigo, dizziness, fatigue, malaise, somnolence.

Pearls: Cost $$$ (≈$1/d retail).
Orthostatic hypotension is common, and many physicians will give the first dose at night.
Prescribe with caution and warn patients of possible hypotensive and orthostatic effects.

One study showed that allowing 2 weeks between dosage changes helped to minimize orthostatic effects.

Pregnancy category B.

DOXORUBICIN (Adriamycin)

Dose: Tumor dependent.

Actions: Cytotoxic anthracycline antibiotic that inhibits synthesis of nucleic acid; used to treat malignancies.

Clearance: 40–50% excreted in bile; minimal renal excretion.

Slightly reduce dosage in ESRD; no change needed for milder renal impairment.

Clearance is reduced in liver dysfunction; adjust dosage based on serum bilirubin: for levels of 1.2–3.0 mg/dL, give 1/2 the normal dose; for levels >3.0 mg/dL, give 1/4 the normal dose.

Side Effects: Cardiotoxicity, leukopenia, frequent nausea and vomiting, reversible alopecia, mucositis (5–10 days after therapy). *Severe* soft tissue injury with possible necrosis can occur if it is extravasated during administration.

Drug Interactions: Can increase hepatotoxicity of 6 mercaptopurine. Can exacerbate cyclophosphamide-induced hemorrhagic cystitis. Concomitant use with cytarabine can cause necrotizing colitis.

Pearls: Cost $$$ (20 mg ≈$100 wholesale).

Cardiotoxicity is the major toxicity. *PDR* recommends obtaining a baseline ECG and repeating after 300 mg/m².

ECG changes include T-wave flattening, ST depression, and arrhythmias, and can last up to 2 weeks after treatment; these changes generally are *not* considered an indication to discontinue therapy.

Life-threatening arrhythmias can occur during or within a few hours after therapy.

Significant LV failure is uncommon but can occur, especially in patients receiving >400–550 mg/m², mediastinal radiation therapy, or concomitant cardiotoxic agents.

Use extreme care to prevent extravasation during administration.

Pregnancy category not established.

DOXYCYCLINE (Vibramycin, Vibra-Tabs)

Dose: Route dependent.
PO: 100 mg bid on day 1, then 100 mg PO qd–bid for at least 6 more days for most infections; may be given without regard to meals, but GI side effects may decrease when taken with food.
IV: 100 mg IV q12h.

Preparations: 50 and 100 mg capsules, 50 and 100 mg tablets; 50 mg/5 mL (1 tsp) syrup; 25 mg/5 mL powder for oral suspension; 100 and 200 mg vials for injection.

Actions: Broad-spectrum bacteriostatic antibiotic that inhibits protein synthesis. Some gram (+) coverage; some gram (−) coverage; some anaerobic coverage including most *B. fragilis*. Also covers *Mycoplasma, Rickettsia,* and *Chlamydia.*

Clearance: Hepatobiliary and renal excreted.
Slightly increase dosing interval in impaired renal function.
Reduce dosage in liver disease (because of possible nephrotoxic effects).
Supplemental dose not required after HD or PD.

Side Effects: GI distress, photosensitivity, tooth discoloration in children and fetuses, hypersensitivity reactions, erosive esophagitis, dose-related increase in BUN, nephrotoxicity, hepatotoxicity.

Drug Interactions: Prolongs PT in patients taking warfarin. Reduces activity of penicillin (avoid concomitant use). Antacids, bicarbonate, calcium, and iron supplements decrease its absorption.

Pearls: Cost $$ (≈$8/wk retail).
Pregnancy category D.

Dramamine: see DIMENHYDRINATE

DTO: see Deodorized Tincture of Opium

Dulcolax: see BISACODYL

Duragesic: see FENTANYL transdermal system

Duricef: see CEFADROXIL

Dyazide (HYDROCHLOROTHIAZIDE + TRIAMTERENE)

Dose: 1 or 2 capsules PO qod–qD, taken after meals.

Preparations: Each capsule contains 25 mg hydrochlorothiazide and 50 mg triamterene.

Actions: K+-sparing diuretic combination; used to treat hypertension.

Drug Interactions: Can raise serum level of lithium.

Cautions: Contraindicated in preexisting hyperkalemia.

Use with caution in severe liver disease (can precipitate hepatic coma) and in patients taking ACE inhibitors (because of its K+-sparing properties).

Pearls: Cost $$ ($\approx$$0.25/d retail).

Pregnancy category C.

DynaCirc: see ISRADIPINE

Dyrenium: see TRIAMTERENE

ECHOTHIOPHATE IODIDE: see Phospholine Iodide

Ecotrin: see ACETYLSALICYLIC ACID

Elavil: see AMITRIPTYLINE

Eminase: see ANISTREPLASE

E-Mycin: see ERYTHROMYCIN

ENALAPRIL (Vasotec)

Dose: Delivery dependent.

PO: First (test) dose: 2.5–5.0 mg; usual, 5–40 mg qd (often given bid in CHF).

IV: 1.25 mg given over 5 min q6h (0.625 mg q6h in renal failure or for patients taking diuretics).

Preparations: 2.5, 5, 10, and 20 mg tablets; 1 and 2 mL vials containing 1.25 mg/mL.

Actions: ACE inhibitor that causes peripheral dilatation; used to treat CHF and hypertension.

Clearance: Some liver metabolism; primarily renal excreted.
Slightly reduce dosage in impaired renal function.
No change needed for liver disease.

Side Effects: Substantial decrease in BP (especially when used with diuretics), dizziness, angioedema, rare decline in WBCs (increased incidence with chronic renal failure and collagen vascular disease), increased BUN and creatinine, increased K^+ (especially with impaired renal function and K^+-sparing drugs), cough, rash, headache.

Cautions: Contraindicated during second and third trimesters of pregnancy and in patients with preexisting hyperkalemia.

Pearls: Cost $$$ (PO ≈$0.70/d retail, IV $34/d wholesale).
Response is decreased in black patients.
Periodically check CBC, BUN, creatinine, and K^+.
Clinical response usually occurs within 15 min with IV form.
Pregnancy category D.

ENCAINIDE (Enkaid)

Dose: Initial, 25 mg PO q8h (not tid); max, 200–300 mg daily in divided doses.

Preparations: 25, 35, and 50 mg capsules.

Actions: Class Ic antiarrhythmic; used to treat ventricular arrhythmias.

Clearance: Metabolized in >90% of patients to two more active metabolites (ODE and MODE) that are excreted in both urine and feces; remaining 10% of patients are slow metabolizers who excrete unchanged drug primarily via kidneys.
It is unclear whether dosage should be adjusted in hepatic failure (one source suggests it is *not* necessary), but any increases in dosing should be done cautiously.

A lower dosage is recommended in impaired renal function with initial dose reduced to 25 mg PO qd in patients with significant renal failure.

Side Effects: Proarrhythmic effects, CNS effects (including dizziness, headache, abnormal vision, tremor and ataxia, fatigue, memory or speech impairment), metallic taste.

Drug Interactions: Cimetidine raises its serum level.

Cautions: Contraindicated in second- or third-degree AV block or bifascicular block unless a ventricular pacer is in place.

Use with caution in sick sinus syndrome.

Pearls: Cost $$$$ (>$2/d retail).

Increases the QRS interval (but this should *not* be used to guide therapy).

The CAST study suggests an increased incidence of adverse events in certain post-MI patients.

Pregnancy category B.

Enkaid: *see* ENCAINIDE

ENTERIC COATED ASPIRIN: *see* ACETYLSALICYLIC ACID

Epifrin: *see* EPINEPHRINE eye drops

EPINEPHRINE

Dose: Route and disease dependent.

Status asthmaticus (in patients <30 years old) and anaphylaxis: IV, 0.3–0.5 mg of 1:10,000 solution; may repeat q5–10min. IM, 0.3–0.5 mg of 1:1,000 solution SQ; may repeat q20–30min up to 3 doses.

Cardiopulmonary resuscitation: 0.5–1.0 mg of 1:10,000 solution IV; may be repeated q5min; may be given down ET tube if no IV access is available.

Actions: Sympathomimetic that directly stimulates α-and β-receptors; used to treat cardiac arrest, status asthmaticus, and anaphylaxis.

Side Effects: Tachyarrhythmias, elevated BP, tremor, headache, anxiety, necrosis of injection site.

Drug Interactions: Tricyclics and MAOI can potentiate its effects.

Cautions: Use with caution in cardiac disease.

Usually is not given to asthmatics >30 years old (because of concerns about possible cardiac disease).

Pearls: Pregnancy category C.

EPINEPHRINE eye drops (Epifrin, Epitrate, Glaucon)

Dose: 1 or 2 drops (written "gtt") bid of 0.5–1.0% solution (packaged as epinephrine borate sodium) or 1 or 2 drops bid of 0.5–2.0% solution (packaged as epinephrine hydrochloride).

Actions: Adrenergic agent; used to treat open-angle glaucoma.

Side Effects (local): Blurred vision, headache, eye irritation, lacrimation.

Side Effects (systemic): A single drop of 2% solution contains 0.1–0.2 mg epinephrine, and some systemic absorption is possible. Systemic reactions can include bronchodilatation, headache, tremor, restlessness, tachycardia, elevated BP, and arrhythmias.

Pearls: Pregnancy category C.

Epitrate: see EPINEPHRINE eye drops

Epogen: see ERYTHROPOIETIN

Erycette: see ERYTHROMYCIN topical solution

Eryderm: see ERYTHROMYCIN topical solution

Erygel: see ERYTHROMYCIN topical gel

Erymax: see ERYTHROMYCIN topical solution

EryPed: see ERYTHROMYCIN ETHYLSUCCINATE

Ery-Tab: see ERYTHROMYCIN

Erythrocin: *see* **ERYTHROMYCIN**

ERYTHROMYCIN (E-Mycin, Ery-Tab, Erythrocin, PCE 333, PCE 500; *see also* Benzamycin, ERYTHROMYCIN ETHYLSUCCINATE)

Dose: Route dependent.

PO: 250 mg qid, or 333 mg tid, or 500 mg bid–qid; PCE 500 is given bid. Generic form should be taken on an empty stomach; E-Mycin, Ery-Tab, and PCE may be taken without regard to meals.

IV: 500 mg–1 g q6h.

Preparations: 250, 333, and 500 mg generic tablets; 250 and 333 mg tablets of E-Mycin; 250, 333, and 500 mg tablets of Ery-Tabs; 333 and 500 mg particle-containing tablets of PCE; 250, 500, and 1000 mg powder preparations for injection.

Actions: Bacteriostatic macrolide antibiotic that reversibly inhibits protein synthesis. Moderate gram (+) coverage including strep and some staph (but *not* MRSA or enterococci). Is drug of choice for *Legionella* and *Mycoplasma*.

Clearance: Excreted via liver into bile.

Slightly reduce dosage in ESRD; no change needed for milder renal impairment.

Use with caution in mild liver dysfunction; decrease dosage for moderate to severe liver disease.

Supplemental dose not required after HD or PD.

Side Effects: Extremely common GI symptoms (abdominal discomfort and cramping, nausea and vomiting, diarrhea), elevated LFTs, mild allergic reaction, transient hearing loss with high doses.

Drug Interactions: Can raise serum level of theophylline. Prolongs PT in patients taking warfarin. Can cause lethal arrhythmias when taken with terfenadine (seldane).

Pearls: Cost: generic $$, PCE $$$ (regular tablets ≈$1/d retail, PCE 333 ≈$3/d retail, PCE 500 ≈$2/d retail).

When given by peripheral IV, phlebitis is common.

GI side effects are associated with IV as well as PO dosing.

The heavy sodium load in the IV preparation may complicate fluid management in critically ill patients.

Pregnancy category not established.

ERYTHROMYCIN ETHYLSUCCINATE (EryPed)

Dose: Pediatric: Weight dependent; suggested usual doses:
Children 10–15 lb, 50 mg PO qid; 16–25 lb, 100 mg PO qid; 26–50 lb, 200 mg PO qid; 51–100 lb, 300 mg PO qid; >100 lb, 400 mg PO qid.

Should be given in 4 equally divided doses; may be given without regard to meals.

Note that because it is an ethylsuccinate preparation, recommended doses are higher than for other erythromycin preparations (which consist of erythromycin as a free base).

Preparations: 200 mg chewable fruit-flavored tablets (EryPed Chewable); 5, 100, and 200 mL bottles of 200 mg/5 mL (1 tsp) suspension (EryPed 200); 5, 60, 100, and 200 mL bottles of 400 mg/5 mL (1 tsp) suspension (EryPed 400).

Actions: Bacteriostatic macrolide antibiotic that reversibly inhibits protein synthesis. Moderate gram (+) coverage including strep and some staph (but *not* MRSA or enterococci). Is drug of choice for *Legionella* and *Mycoplasma*.

Clearance: Excreted via liver into bile.

Slightly reduce dosage in ESRD; no change needed for milder renal impairment.

Use with caution in mild liver dysfunction; decrease dosage in moderate to severe liver disease.

Supplemental dose not required after HD or PD.

Side Effects: Extremely common GI symptoms (abdominal discomfort and cramping, nausea and vomiting, diarrhea), elevated LFTs, mild allergic reaction, transient hearing loss with high doses.

Drug Interactions: Can raise serum level of theophylline. Prolongs PT in patients taking warfarin.

Pearls: Cost $$$.

ERYTHROMYCIN ophthalmic ointment (Ilotycin)

Dose: Apply to infected structure qd or more frequently.

Preparations: 1/8 oz tube containing 0.5% erythromycin.

Actions: Topical antibiotic; used to treat corneal and conjunctival infections.

Pearls: Cost $$ (1/8 oz tube: generic ≈$5; Ilotycin ≈$8).
Pregnancy category B.

ERYTHROMYCIN topical solution and gel (Erycette, Eryderm, Erygel, Erymax)

Dose: Apply to cleansed, dried skin bid.

Preparations: All contain 2% erythromycin. Erycette solution available in boxes containing 60 individual-dose swabs; Eryderm solution available in 60 mL bottles with applicator; Erygel cream available in 30 and 60 g plastic tubes; Erymax solution available in 2 and 4 oz bottles.

Actions: Topical antibiotic; used to treat acne vulgaris.

Pearls: Cost: generic $$, brands $$$ (generic ≈$10 retail per bottle, brands ≈$20 retail per bottle or tube).
Pregnancy category not established.

ERYTHROPOIETIN (Epogen)

Dose: Initial, 50–100 units/kg given 3 times a week, IV for dialysis patients, IV or SQ for patients with chronic renal failure who are not on dialysis; maintenance, highly individualized.

Some physicians will begin with a lower initial dose of 20–40 units/kg (in part for financial and reimbursement reasons).

Decrease dosage when target hematocrit is reached or if hematocrit increases >4% in any 2-week period.

Preparations: 2000, 4000, and 10,000 unit injection.

Actions: Recombinant human glycoprotein that stimulates RBC production; used to treat anemia in chronic renal failure.

Side Effects: Elevated BP (especially after initial therapy), increased seizures, transient rash, headache, arthralgias, iron defiency, thrombocytosis, diaphoresis.

Cautions: Contraindicated in patients with uncontrolled hypertension or with hypersensitivity to human albumin or mammalian cell-derived products.

Pearls: Cost $$$$ (40 units/kg $\approx$$100/wk wholesale).
Check hematocrit twice weekly.
Check iron stores before beginning treatment and follow them periodically.
Reticulocyte count should increase within 10 days and hematocrit within 2–6 weeks; rate of hematocrit increase is dose dependent.
Serum erythropoietin level is 0.01–0.03 units/mL in normal subjects and can increase 100- to 1000-fold during hypoxemia or anemia.
Pregnancy category C.

Esgic (BUTALBITAL, ACETAMINOPHEN + CAFFEINE)

Dose: 1 or 2 capsules or tablets PO q4h prn; max, 6 capsules or tablets in 24 h.

Preparations: Each capsule or tablet contains 50 mg butalbital, 40 mg caffeine, and 325 mg acetaminophen.

Pearls: Cost: generic $$$, Esgic $$$$ (generic $\approx$$1/d retail, Esgic $\approx$$2.50/d retail).
Is chemically similar to Fioricet.
Pregnancy category not established.

ESMOLOL (Brevibloc)

Dose: Loading: 500 μg/kg over 1 min, then give 50 μg/kg/min for 4 min; may repeat loading dose and increase maintenance dose by 50 μg/kg/min q5min.
Most patients respond to infusion rate of 150–200 μg/kg/min; may then gradually reduce infusion rate.

Preparations: 10 mL vial containing 10 mg/mL ready for injection; 10 mL ampule containing 2.5 g of drug that must be diluted before injection.

Actions: Ultra-short-acting β_1-selective β-blocker; used for acute treatment of angina, arrhythmias, and other conditions.

Clearance: Metabolized by esterase in RBCs; $t_{1/2}$ is 9 min.

Side Effects: Substantially reduced BP, increased risk of CHF, nausea and vomiting, syncope, angina, AV block, bronchospasm.

Drug Interactions: Raises serum level of digoxin by 10–20%. Morphine raises its serum level 46%.

Pearls: Cost $$$$ ($\approx$$100/d wholesale, 10 mL vial $\approx$$1 wholesale).
Pregnancy category C.

ESTAZOLAM (ProSom)

Dose: Initial, 1–2 mg PO qhs prn; consider beginning with 0.5 mg in small, debilitated, or elderly patients.

Preparations: 1 and 2 mg scored tablets.

Actions: Benzodiazepine; used to treat insomnia.

Side Effects: Somnolence and sedation, hypokinesia, dizziness, abnormal coordination.

Cautions: Should not be used in pregnant or potentially pregnant patients.

Pearls: Cost $$ ($\approx$$0.60/d retail).
Abrupt discontinuance can cause rebound insomnia.
Was given a relatively negative review by *The Medical Letter* [33:854, Oct 4 1991].
Pregnancy category X.

ESTROGEN: see Premarin

ETHAMBUTOL

Dose: Usual, 15 mg/kg PO qd; some sources recommend giving 25 mg/kg PO qd for first 2 months of treatment, or initially for severe infections.

Preparations: 100 and 400 mg tablets.

Actions: Bacteriostatic antitubercular agent that inhibits metabolite synthesis; used to treat mycobacterial infections.

Clearance: Some excretion in feces; primarily renal excreted.
Slightly to moderately increase dosing interval in impaired renal function.
No change in dosage needed for liver disease.
Supplemental dose suggested after HD or PD.

Side Effects: Decreased visual acuity (from optic neuritis), elevated uric acid levels, rare peripheral neuropathy.

Cautions: Contraindicated in optic neuritis.

Pearls: Cost $$$1/2 (≈$2/d retail).
Initial visual check is prudent; some sources recommend regular visual examinations.
Pregnancy category not established.

ETHINYL ESTRADIOL: see Norinyl, Ortho-Novum, TriLevlen, Tri-Norinyl, Triphasil oral contraceptive pills

Ethmozine: see MORICIZINE

ETHOSUXIMIDE (Zarontin)

Dose: Initial, 250 mg PO bid; may increase by 250 mg daily (not bid) every 4–7 days until effective. Max, 1.5 g daily. Usual maintenance, 10–20 mg/kg PO bid.

Preparations: 250 mg capsules; 50 mg/mL syrup.

Actions: Succinimide anticonvulsant; used to treat petit-mal seizures.

Clearance: Primarily metabolized; some renal excretion.
Slightly reduce dosage in ESRD; no change needed for mild renal impairment.
No change in dosage needed for liver disease.
Supplemental dose suggested after HD.

Side Effects: GI distress, nausea and vomiting, anorexia and weight loss.

Pearls: Cost $$$$ (≈$4/d retail).

Has been reported to cause leukopenia (rarely), SLE, aplastic anemia, and Stevens-Johnson syndrome.

Although other anticonvulsants have been shown to cause birth defects, the risks of ethosuximide during pregnancy have not been clearly established. Risks of continuing therapy must be weighed against the risk of seizures during pregnancy.

ETODOLAC (Lodine)

Dose: 200 mg PO tid–qid, or 300 mg PO bid–qid, or 400 mg PO bid–tid.

Preparations: 200 and 300 mg capsules.

Actions: NSAID; used to treat osteoarthritis and mild to moderate pain.

Side Effects: Dyspepsia, upper GI bleeding, fluid retention. Theoretical worsening of "prerenal" renal failure.

Cautions: Contraindicated in allergy to ASA or other NSAID. Use with extreme caution, if at all, in patients with history of upper GI bleeding or ulcer disease. Use with caution in renal disease.

Pearls: Cost $$$$ (≈$2.70/d retail).

Pregnancy category C.

ETOPOSIDE (VePesid, VP-16)

Dose: Variable; may be given PO or IV.

Frequent IV regimen: 35–100 mg/m$_2$/d for 5 consecutive days or 100 mg/m$_2$ on days 1, 3, and 5.

Preparations: 50 mg capsules; 100 mg/5 mL vials for injection.

Actions: Cell-cycle-specific semisynthetic derivative of podophyllotoxin, a plant resin with cathartic and antineoplastic properties; used to treat neoplasms.

Clearance: Undergoes some metabolism, biliary excretion (16%), and urinary excretion (30–40%).

Slightly reduce dosage in impaired renal function.

Side Effects: Anaphylactic reaction, decreased WBCs and platelets, nausea and vomiting, reversible alopecia.

Cautions: Give slowly (over 30–60 min) to avoid hypotension.

Pearls: Cost $$$ (100 mg $117 wholesale).

Bone marrow suppression is dose-limiting toxicity.

Follow CBC.

Granulocyte nadir occurs in 7–14 days, and platelet nadir in 9–16 days.

Bone marrow recovery is usually complete by day 20.

Pregnancy category D.

Ex-Lax (unflavored), Ex-Lax Chocolate laxative, Extra Gentle Ex-Lax

Dose: 1 or 2 pills with water qhs.

Preparations: Boxes of 8, 30, and 60 unflavored pills; boxes of 6, 18, 48, and 72 chewable chocolate-flavored tablets; boxes of 24 Extra Gentle Ex-Lax pills.

Actions: Laxative containing active ingredient phenolphthalein; used to treat occasional constipation.

EXPECTORANTS: see GUAIFENESIN

FAMOTIDINE (Pepcid)

Dose: Situation dependent.

Acute therapy: 20 mg IV q12h or 40 mg PO qhs for 4–8 weeks.

Maintenance therapy: 20 mg PO qhs.

Preparations: 20 and 40 mg tablets; 400 mg powder for reconstitution, giving 40 mg/5 mL (1 tsp) oral suspension; 2 and 4 mg vials containing 10 mg/mL for injection.

Actions: H$_2$-blocker; used to treat peptic ulcer disease, gastritis, esophageal reflux, and Zollinger-Ellison syndrome.

Clearance: Mainly renal excreted.
Slightly reduce dosage in impaired renal function.
No change in dosage needed for liver disease.

Side Effects: Headache (rare), dizziness, constipation, diarrhea.

Drug Interactions: Magnesium- and aluminum-containing antacids, such as Maalox and Mylanta, reduce its bioavailability (give at least 2 h apart from it).

Pearls: Cost $$$ (≈$1/d retail).
Pregnancy category B.

Feldene: see PIROXICAM

FELODIPINE (Plendil)

Dose: Initial, 5 mg PO qd; maintenance, 5–20 mg PO qd. Elderly patients may require lower dosage.

Preparations: 5 and 10 mg tablets.

Actions: Calcium-channel blocker that works primarily through peripheral vasodilatation; used to treat hypertension.

Clearance: Metabolized via liver.
No change in dosage needed for impaired renal function.
Reduce dosage in liver disease.

Side Effects: Hypotension, dizziness, peripheral edema, reflex tachycardia, palpitations, headache, flushing.

Drug Interactions: Cimetidine can raise its serum level. Can increase serum level of digoxin.

Pearls: Cost $$$$ (10 mg ≈$170 retail/100 tablets).
Caution patients about possible hypotensive effects.
Has no significant effects on cardiac conductivity.
Studies to date have shown no significant ($-$) inotropic effects.
Pregnancy category C.

FENTANYL transdermal system (Duragesic)

Dose: Initial, 25 μg/h as Duragesic-25 patch applied to skin; change each patch after 3 days' use. Titrate to pain as needed.

Preparations: 25, 50, and 100 μg patches.

Actions: Topical synthetic narcotic; used to treat chronic pain that requires opioid analgesia.

Side Effects: Nausea and vomiting, urine retention, pruritus, hypoventilation, CNS effects.

Pearls: Cost $$$$ (50 μg patch ≈$13 retail each).

New equilibration is reached 6 days after a dosage change, so allow 1 week before increasing dose.

Use a short-acting narcotic during first 24 h to supplement analgesic relief.

Fentanyl is 100 times more potent than morphine.

For total daily PO morphine dose of 45–134 mg, use transdermal fentanyl at 25 μg/h; for 500 mg dose, use fentanyl at 125–150 μg/h; for 1000 mg dose, use fentanyl at 275 μg/h.

Pregnancy category C.

Fergon: see FERROUS GLUCONATE

FERROUS GLUCONATE (Fergon)

Dose: 1 or 2 tablets or 1–2 tsp PO qd.

Preparations: 320 mg tablets containing 38 mg elemental ferrous iron; 1 pint bottles of 6% elixir.

Actions: Iron supplement.

Pearls: Cost $ (≈$4 retail/100 tablets).

May be better tolerated and produce less constipation than ferrous sulfate.

Generally regarded as safe during pregnancy.

FERROUS SULFATE (IRON, FeSO$_4$)

Dose: Route dependent.
PO: 325 mg bid–tid.
Elixir: 1 or 2 tsp tid, preferably between meals.

Preparations: 325 mg tablets; 16 oz bottles of elixir containing 220 mg/5 mL (1 tsp).

Side Effects: Nausea, indigestion, diarrhea, abdominal cramping, constipation.

Pearls: Cost $ ($0.15/d retail).
Taking with meals reduces its GI side effects.
Consider giving with an anticonstipation agent (Colace, Metamucil, etc.).
Turns stools black, which can be misinterpreted as melena.
Most patients do not tolerate tid dosing, and bid dosing is recommended by some physicians for increased compliance.
For those unable to tolerate ferrous sulfate, ferrous citrate (contained in Geritol) or ferrous gluconate may be more palatable alternatives.
Generally regarded as safe during pregnancy.

Fioricet (BUTALBITAL, ACETAMINOPHEN + CAFFEINE)

Dose: 1 or 2 capsules PO q4h prn; max, 6 capsules daily.

Preparations: Each capsule contains 50 mg butalbital, 325 mg acetaminophen, and 40 mg caffeine.

Actions: Medication that combines analgesic properties of acetaminophen and caffeine with anxiolytic and muscle-relaxant properties of butalbital (a barbiturate); usually used to treat migraine headaches.

Side Effects: Drowsiness, dizziness, light-headedness, nausea and vomiting, mental confusion, flatulence.

Drug Interactions: Butalbital increases metabolism of warfarin and decreases serum level of tricyclics. Fioricet potentiates CNS depressant effects of other CNS depressants.

Cautions: Use with caution in liver disease (because of potential hepatotoxicity from acetaminophen) and in patients who must perform potentially hazardous tasks.

Pearls: Cost $$$ (≈$35 retail/100 tablets).
May cause rebound headaches.
Pregnancy category not established.

Fiorinal (BUTALBITAL, ASA + CAFFEINE)

Dose: 1 or 2 capsules or tablets PO q4h prn; max, 6 capsules or tablets daily.

Preparations: Each capsule or tablet contains 50 mg butalbital, 325 mg ASA, and 40 mg caffeine.

Actions: Medication that combines analgesic properties of ASA with anxiolytic and muscle-relaxant properties of butalbital (a barbiturate); usually used to treat migraine headaches.

Side Effects: CNS depression, drowsiness, dizziness, impairment of mental and physical skills, light-headedness, nausea and vomiting, flatulence.

Drug Interactions: Butalbital increases metabolism of warfarin and reduces serum level of tricyclics. Fiorinal potentiates CNS depressant effects of other CNS depressants.

Cautions: Contraindicated in porphyria.
Use with caution in peptic ulcer disease or coagulopathy and in patients who must perform potentially hazardous tasks.

Pearls: Cost $$$ (≈$35 retail/100 tablets).
Pregnancy category not established.

Flagyl: see METRONIDAZOLE

FLECAINIDE (Tambocor)

Dose: Initial, 100 mg PO q12h; max, 400 mg daily (usually given q12h).

Preparations: 50, 100, and 150 mg tablets.

Actions: Class Ic antiarrhythmic; used to treat ventricular arrhythmias.

Clearance: Metabolized via liver; renal excreted.
Slightly reduce dosage in impaired renal function.
Some sources suggest an initial dose of 50 mg PO q12h and lower maintenance doses in chronic renal failure, and lower maintenance doses or increased dosing intervals in liver disease.
Supplemental dose not required after HD.

Side Effects: Proarrhythmic effects, $(-)$ inotropy, CHF, frequent neurologic side effects. Can raise the pacing threshold.

Drug Interactions: Amiodarone can markedly raise its serum level. Cimetidine increases and hepatic enzyme inducers reduce its serum level. Concomitant use with propranolol raises serum levels of both drugs.

Cautions: Contraindicated in second- or third-degree AV block and in bifascicular block unless a ventricular pacer is in place.
Contraindicated in severe CHF.
Use with extreme caution in patients with sick sinus syndrome.

Pearls: Cost $$$$ ($\approx$$2/d retail).
The CAST study suggests an increased incidence of adverse events in certain post-MI patients treated with flecainide.
Should be discontinued only in hospital setting.
Pregnancy category C.

Flexeril: see CYCLOBENZAPRINE

Florinef: see FLUDROCORTISONE

Floxin: see OFLOXACIN

FLUCONAZOLE (Diflucan)

Dose: Disease dependent.
Oropharyngeal or esophageal candidiasis: 200 mg "loading dose" PO or IV, then 100 mg PO or IV qd for 2–3 weeks.
Systemic candidiasis or acute cryptococcal meningitis: 400 mg "loading dose" PO or IV, then 200 mg PO or IV qd for 10–12 weeks.

Preparations: 100 and 200 mg tablets.

Actions: Antifungal antibiotic; used to treat local or systemic candidiasis and cryptococcal meningitis.

Clearance: Primarily renal excreted; some excretion in feces.
Moderately reduce dosage in impaired renal function.
No change in dosage needed for liver disease.

Side Effects: Nausea and vomiting, headache, skin rash, abdominal pain and diarrhea. May cause rare elevation in LFTs.

Drug Interactions: Raises serum level of phenytoin. Reduces metabolism and raises serum level of OHAs. Prolongs PT in patients taking warfarin. Infrequently raises serum level of cyclosporine. Rifampin increases its metabolism.

Pearls: Cost $$$$ (PO ≈$90 retail/2 wk of therapy, 200 mg IV injection ≈$100).
Watch patients for symptoms and signs of hepatic injury; follow LFTs.
Pregnancy category C.

FLUDROCORTISONE (Florinef)

Dose: Range, 0.05–0.2 mg (50–200 μg) PO qd; usual, 50 μg PO qd–qod.

Preparations: 0.1 mg (100 μg) tablets.

Actions: Oral cortisol derivative with potent mineralocorticoid and moderate glucocorticoid effects; used to treat adrenocortical insufficiency.

Side Effects: Hypertension, edema, weight gain, CHF, hypernatremia, hypokalemia, cardiac hypertrophy.

Pearls: Cost $$ (0.1 mg generic $30 wholesale/100 tablets).

FLUOCINONIDE cream, gel, ointment, and solution (Lidex)

Dose: Apply thin film to affected skin bid–qid.

Preparations: 15, 30, 60, and 120 g 0.05% cream; 15, 30, 60, and 120 g 0.05% gel; 15, 30, 60, and 120 g 0.05% ointment; 20 and 60 mL 0.05% solution.

Actions: Topical steroid; used to treat steroid-responsive dermatologic conditions.

Side Effects: Local irritation, dermatitis, folliculitis, hypertrichosis, adrenal axis suppression.

Cautions: Contraindicated in varicella or vaccinia.

Pearls: Cost: generic $$, Lidex $$$ (60 g retail: generic ≈$20, Lidex ≈$40).
  Pregnancy category C.

FLUOROMETHOLONE ophthalmic ointment and suspension (FML, FML Forte)

Dose: Delivery dependent.
  Suspension: Instill 1 drop (written "gtt") bid–qid.
  Ointment: Apply 0.5-inch "ribbon" qd–tid.

Preparations: 3.5 g tube of FML ointment containing 0.1% fluorometholone; 1, 5, 10, and 15 mL suspensions of FML containing 0.1% fluorometholone; 2, 5, 10, and 15 mL suspensions of FML Forte containing 0.25% fluorometholone.

Actions: Topical corticosteroid; used to treat inflammatory conditions.

Cautions: Contraindicated in possible herpes simplex infection.

Pearls: Pregnancy category C.

5-FLUOROURACIL (5-FU)

Dose: Tumor dependent. Often 12 mg/kg/d IV for 4 days, then 6 mg/kg IV on days 6, 8, 10, and 12 if no toxicity develops.

Actions: Antineoplastic antimetabolite that interferes with DNA and RNA synthesis; used to treat malignancies.

Clearance: Metabolized primarily via liver; 7%–20% renal excreted.

No change in dosage needed for impaired renal function.

Use with caution in liver disease.

Side Effects: Stomatitis and esophagopharyngitis, anorexia, nausea and vomiting, diarrhea, dermatitis, pruritus, transient alopecia, decreased WBCs.

Drug Interactions: Leukovorin can enhance its toxicity.

Cautions: Contraindicated in patients with poor nutritional status, depressed bone marrow function, or serious infections.

Pearls: Cost $ (1 g ≈$8 wholesale).

PDR recommends discontinuing therapy in patients with WBCs <3500 or rapidly falling WBC count, intractable vomiting or diarrhea, GI ulceration and bleeding, platelets <100,000, or clinical bleeding.

WBC nadir generally occurs on days 9–14 and WBCs usually return to normal by day 30.

Pregnancy category D.

FLUOXETINE (Prozac)

Dose: Initial, 20 mg PO qd; max, 80 mg daily (given 40 mg PO bid).

Preparations: 20 mg capsules; 20 mg/5 mL (1 tsp) liquid.

Actions: Nontricyclic agent that probably inhibits serotonin reuptake; used to treat depression.

Clearance: Metabolized via liver.

PDR recommends reducing dosage in severe renal disease.

$t_{1/2}$ is increased in liver disease, so dosage adjustment may be needed.

Side Effects: Tremor, anxiety, nervousness, insomnia, akathisia, sexual dysfunction, abnormal dreams, sweating, GI complaints, altered appetite, weight loss, rash or urticaria, SIADH, hyponatremia.

Drug Interactions: Can prolong $t_{1/2}$ of concurrently administered benzodiazepines. Increases plasma levels of concurrently administered antidepressants. Severe reactions with MAOI.

Cautions: Contraindicated in patients taking MAOI.

Pearls: Cost $$$$ ($\approx$$2/capsule retail).
   Allow 14 days after discontinuance of MAOI before beginning therapy.
   Allow 5 weeks after discontinuance of Prozac before beginning MAOI.
   Pregnancy category B.

FLURAZEPAM (Dalmane)

Dose: 15–30 mg PO qhs prn.

Preparations: 15 and 30 mg capsules.

Actions: Long-acting benzodiazepine; used to treat insomnia.

Clearance: Metabolized via liver.
   No change in dosage needed for impaired renal function.
   One source recommends reducing dosage in liver disease.

Side Effects: Post-dose daytime hangover.

Cautions: Should not be used in pregnant or potentially pregnant patients.

Pearls: Cost: generic $, Dalmane $$$ (generic $\approx$$18 retail/100 tablets, 100 mg Dalmane $\approx$$56 retail); costs of 15 mg and 30 mg capsules are similar.
   May cause excessive drowsiness in elderly patients.
   Contraindicated during pregnancy.

FML, FML Forte: see FLUOROMETHOLONE ophthalmic ointment and suspension

FOLIC ACID

Dose: 1 mg PO qd for 2–3 weeks.
Some patients may need chronic replacement therapy.

Preparations: 0.1, 0.4, 0.8, and 1.0 mg tablets; 5 and 10 mg/mL for injection.

Pearls: Cost $ (≈$3.50 retail/100 tablets).

May prevent dysplasia of colonic epithelium in ulcerative colitis when given as therapy with sulfasalazine (Azulfidine).

In patients who are NPO (such as alcoholics with pancreatitis), folate may be given IV by adding 1 mg of folate to the hanging IV fluid.

Generally regarded as safe during pregnancy.

Fortaz: *see* CEFTAZIDIME

FOSINOPRIL (Monopril)

Dose: Initial, 10 mg PO qd; maintenance, 20–40 mg PO qd.

Preparations: 10 and 20 mg tablets.

Actions: ACE inhibitor pro-drug; used to treat hypertension.

Clearance: Metabolized via liver; excreted equally in feces and urine.

No change in dosage needed for impaired renal function.

Is poorly dialyzed.

Dosage adjustment generally not required in elderly patients.

Side Effects: Cough, dizziness and hypotension, angioedema, hyperkalemia, possible worsening of "prerenal" renal failure.

Cautions: Contraindicated during second and third trimesters of pregnancy and in patients who have experienced angioedema with other ACE inhibitors.

Pearls: Cost $$ (≈$0.70/d retail).

Caution patients about possible hypotensive effects and angioedema.

Follow K^+, BUN, and creatinine.

Periodically check WBCs (another ACE inhibitor has been associated with rare neutropenia).

Absorption is not affected by food.

Pregnancy category D.

5-FU: *see* 5-FLUOROURACIL

Fulvicin P/G, Fulvicin-U/F: *see* GRISEOFULVIN

FUROSEMIDE (Lasix)

Dose: Initial, 10–20 mg PO or IV; max, 600 mg daily. Usually no more than 400 mg is given at any one time.

Preparations: 20, 40, and 80 mg tablets; 10 mg/mL and 40 mg/5 mL solution; 5 and 10 mg/mL injection.

Actions: Loop diuretic that causes early increase in venodilation and later diuresis; used to treat CHF and edema.

Clearance: Some liver metabolism; primarily renal excreted.

No change in dosage needed for impaired renal function.

May need to reduce dosage in liver disease.

Side Effects: Decreased K^+ and Na^+, substantially reduced BP, hypochloremic alkalosis, ototoxicity (especially when injected too rapidly). Can increase ototoxicity of aminoglycosides. Can raise serum glucose level.

Pearls: Cost $ (100 tablets retail: 20 mg PO generic ≈$8, 20 mg PO Lasix ≈$14; 80 mg IV ≈$1).

Inject slowly (<20 mg/min) to minimize ototoxicity.

Concomitant use of metolazone (Zaroxolyn) or chlorothiazide (Diuril) can potentiate its effect.

PO peak diuretic effect occurs at 1–2 h; duration of effect 6–8 h.

IV peak diuretic effect occurs at 30 min; duration of effect 2 h.

Pregnancy category C.

Garamycin: *see* GENTAMICIN

Garamycin Ophthalmic: *see* GENTAMICIN SULFATE eye drops

Gas-X: *see* SIMETHICONE

G-CSF: *see* GRANULOCYTE COLONY-STIMULATING FACTOR

GEMFIBROZIL (Lopid)

Dose: 600 mg PO bid given 30 min before meals.

Preparations: 600 mg tablets; 300 mg capsules.

Actions: Fibric acid derivative that inhibits hepatic triglyceride synthesis, leading to reduced VLDL and triglycerides, increased HDL, and increased or decreased LDL; used to treat hypercholesterolemia and hypertriglyceridemia.

Clearance: Metabolized via liver; renal excreted.
Moderately reduce dosage in impaired renal function.

Side Effects: Dyspepsia, abdominal pain, flatulence, gallbladder disease, rare elevated LFTs, rare decrease in CBC, skin reactions. Can cause cataracts.

Drug Interactions: Can cause rhabdomyolysis if given with lovastatin (Mevacor).

Cautions: Contraindicated in hepatic or gallbladder disease, in severe renal dysfunction, and in patients taking lovastatin.
Probably should also not be used concurrently with other HMG-CoA inhibitors such as Simvastatin (Zocor) and Pravastatin (Pravachol).

Pearls: Cost $$$$ ($\approx$$2/d retail).
Pregnancy category B.

Genoptic: *see* GENTAMICIN SULFATE eye drops

GENTAMICIN (Garamycin)

Dose: Loading, 2 mg/kg; maintenance, 1–1.67 mg/kg q8h IM or IV.

Preparations: 2 mL vials containing 40 mg/mL for injection.

Actions: Bactericidal aminoglycoside antibiotic that irreversibly inhibits protein synthesis. Excellent aerobic gram (−) coverage including some *P. aeruginosa* (in some institutions, hospital-acquired *Pseudomonas* infections may be resistant). May be used with a penicillin, cephalosporin, or vancomycin for synergy against staph, strep, and enterococci; *not* effective against anaerobes.

Clearance: Renal excreted.
Markedly reduce dosage or increase dosing interval in impaired renal function.
No change in dosage needed for liver disease.
Supplemental dose suggested after HD or PD.

Side Effects: Nephrotoxicity, ototoxicity, fever. Can increase neuromuscular blockade.

Drug Interactions: Some cephalosporins, vancomycin, loop diuretics, cisplatin, and cyclosporin increase risk of nephrotoxicity or ototoxicity.

Pearls: Cost $ (≈$10/d wholesale); significantly less expensive than amikacin or tobramycin.
No significant CSF penetration.
Can be administered intrathecally.
Follow serum peak and trough levels. Each hospital and source has different peak and slightly different trough ranges; reasonable generalizations are peak levels 5–10 μg/mL and trough levels <2–4 μg/mL, but *each hospital's guidelines must be followed*.
Pregnancy category not established.

GENTAMICIN SULFATE eye drops (Garamycin Ophthalmic, Genoptic)

Dose: 1 or 2 drops (written "gtt") q4h; in severe infections may give up to 2 drops hourly (as directed by an ophthalmologist).

Preparations: 3.5 g ointment containing 0.3% gentamicin; 5 mL solution containing 0.3% gentamicin.

Actions: Antibiotic eye drop.

Pearls: Cost $$ (≈$10–12 retail).
Watch for toxicity from systemic absorption.
Pregnancy category C.

Glaucon: see EPINEPHRINE eye drops

GLIPIZIDE (Glucotrol)

Dose: Initial, 5 mg PO qd (2.5 mg in elderly patients and patients with liver dysfunction); max, 40 mg daily. Give bid if >15 mg daily.

Preparations: 5 and 10 mg tablets.

Actions: Oral hypoglycemic of sulfonylurea group; used to treat non-insulin-dependent diabetes.

Clearance: Metabolized via liver.
No change in dosage needed for impaired renal function.
Initial dose in patients with liver disease should be 2.5 mg PO qd.

Side Effects: Hypoglycemia, nausea, diarrhea, constipation, allergic skin reaction, elevated LFTs, rare decrease in CBC or hyponatremia.

Drug Interactions: Hypoglycemia is increased with other sulfonylureas, insulin, ASA, NSAID, sulfonamides, warfarin, MAOI, and β-blockers. Hyperglycemia is increased with diuretics, steroids, thyroid hormone, phenothiazines, phenytoin, nicotinic acid, sympathomimetics, isoniazid, and calcium-channel blockers.

Pearls: Cost $$$ (≈$1/d retail); tolbutamide is significantly less expensive.
Give 30 min before a meal.
Signs and symptoms of hypoglycemia can be masked in elderly patients and in patients taking β-blockers.
Duration of action is 12–18 h.
Increased hypoglycemia is more common in elderly debilitated patients or patients with renal, hepatic, adrenal, or pituitary impairment, in alcohol use, and in severe or prolonged exercise.
Increased hyperglycemia is more common with fever, trauma, infection, surgery, or other types of stress.
Pregnancy category C.

GLUCAGON

Dose: 1 mg (1 unit) IM or SQ.

Preparations: 1 mg (1 unit) vial with 1 mL of diluting solution; 10 mg (10 unit) vial with 10 mL of diluting solution.

Actions: Pancreatic hormone that causes the liver to release glucose into the bloodstream; used to replenish serum levels of glucose in hypoglycemic patients when IV access to inject glucose directly is not available.

Side Effects: Nausea and vomiting, rash or allergic reactions.

Pearls: Useful only in patients with adequate liver stores of glycogen.
   Can cause a pheochromocytoma to release catecholamines.
   Do not combine with normal saline while injecting.

Glucotrol: see GLIPIZIDE

GLYBURIDE (DiaBeta, Micronase)

Dose: Initial, 2.5–5.0 mg PO qd (1.25 mg in more sensitive patients); max, 20 mg daily, usually given as 10 mg bid.

Preparations: 1.25, 2.5, and 5 mg tablets.

Actions: Oral hypoglycemic of sulfonylurea group; used to treat non-insulin-dependent diabetes.

Clearance: Metabolized via liver.
   No change in dosage needed for impaired renal function.

Side Effects: Hypoglycemia, elevated LFTs, hepatitis, cholestatic jaundice, allergic skin reaction, rare reduction in CBC or Na^+.

Drug Interactions: Increased hypoglycemia with other sulfonylureas, insulin, ASA, NSAID, sulfonamides, warfarin, MAOI, and β-blockers. Increased hyperglycemia with diuretics, steroids, thyroid hormone, phenothiazines, phenytoin, nicotinic acid, sympathomimetic drugs, isoniazid, and calcium-channel blockers.

Pearls: Cost $$$ (≈$1/d retail); tolbutamide is significantly less expensive.

Give with morning meal.

Effectiveness decreases in many patients over time.

Increases hypoglycemia in elderly, debilitated, or malnourished patients and in patients with renal, hepatic, adrenal, or pituitary impairment, in alcohol use, and in severe or prolonged exercise.

Signs and symptoms of hypoglycemia can be masked in elderly patients and in patients taking β-blockers.

Pregnancy category B.

GLYCERIN suppository

Dose: 1 suppository (2.7 g) PR.

Actions: Laxative.

Pearls: Onset of action is 2–60 min. Should be retained in colon for 15–20 min.

GLYCEROL, IODINATED: see Organidin

GLYCOPYRROLATE (Robinul)

Dose: 1 mg PO tid or 2 mg PO bid–tid.

Preparations: 1 and 2 mg tablets.

Actions: Anticholinergic agent; used to treat peptic ulcer disease, diarrhea, and reactive airway disease.

Side Effects: Drowsiness, blurred vision, tachycardia, mydriasis, heat prostration.

Cautions: Contraindicated in glaucoma, obstructive uropathy, obstructive GI tract disease, paralytic ileus, severe ulcerative colitis, toxic megacolon, and myasthenia gravis.

Use with caution in elderly patients and in patients with autonomic neuropathy, hepatic or renal disease, ulcerative colitis, hiatal hernia with reflux esophagitis, CAD, CHF, or hyperthyroidism.

Pearls: Cost $$ ($\approx$$0.50/d retail).
Also available in parenteral form (given at lower doses).
Pregnancy category not established.

GM-CSF: see GRANULOCYTE-MACROPHAGE COLONY-STIMULATING FACTOR

GoLYTELY (POLYETHYLENE GLYCOL–ELECTROLYE SOLUTION)

Dose: 4 liters (yes, liters!) PO over several hours.

Preparations: 4 liter jugs containing powder for reconstitution with water.

Actions: Nonabsorbable osmotic agent; used for bowel preparation before GI examinations.

Side Effects: Nausea, bloating, cramps, vomiting.

Cautions: Contraindicated in suspected GI obstruction or perforation.

Pearls: Must aggressively encourage patients to consume 4 liters.
Pregnancy category C.

GRANULOCYTE COLONY-STIMULATING FACTOR (G-CSF, Neupogen)

Dose: Initial, 5 μg/kg/d SQ or IV; may increase in 5 μg/kg increments.

Actions: Hematopoietic growth factor that promotes proliferation, maturation, and migration of neutrophils; used to decrease the incidence of infections in patients with chemotherapy-related neutropenia.

Side Effects: Gout, bone pain, exacerbation of psoriasis, increased alkaline phosphatase and lactate dehydrogenase, proliferation of several tumor lines.

Pearls: Cost $$$$.

Neutrophil counts achieve and maintain a plateau on day 3 of treatment.

Neutrophil counts increase sixfold within 5 days of starting treatment and decrease by 50% within 2 days of discontinuance.

Several clinical differences exist between G-CSF and GM-CSF.

GRANULOCYTE-MACROPHAGE COLONY-STIMULATING FACTOR (GM-CSF, Prokine, Sargramostim)

Dose: 250 µg/m²/d, given over 2 h, each day for 21 days after autologous bone marrow transplantation.

Preparations: 500 µg vials for reconstitution.

Actions: Recombinant DNA–produced glycoprotein that stimulates proliferation and differentiation of hematopoietic progenitor cells; used to treat patients following bone marrow transplantation.

Side Effects: Generally well tolerated: most side effects were no more common in treatment group than in placebo group. Watch for peripheral edema, pleural or pericardial effusion, dyspnea (from sequestration of granulocytes in pulmonary circulation), transient SVT.

Pearls: Follow CBC and differential twice weekly.

In vitro activity includes stimulating proliferation or differentiation of progenitor cells; stimulating maturation cycle of neutrophils, monocytes or macrophages, and eosinophils; and increasing function of mature neutrophils and monocytes or macrophages.

Clinical effects in bone marrow transplant recipients include modest shortening of hospital stay, reduced duration of neutropenia, and possible decrease in infections and need for antibiotics.

Treatment did not improve 1-year survival when compared with placebo.

Pregnancy category C.

Grifulvin V: see GRISEOFULVIN

Grisactin, Grisactin Ultra: *see* **GRISEOFULVIN**

GRISEOFULVIN (Fulvicin P/G, Fulvicin-U/F, Grifulvin V, Grisactin, Grisactin Ultra)

Dose: Delivery dependent.
Griseofulvin microsize: 500 mg PO qd or 500 mg PO bid.
Griseofulvin ultramicrosize: 330 mg PO qd or 330 mg PO bid.
Griseofulvin ultramicrosize is more completely absorbed than griseofulvin microsize, so daily dose can be 1/3 less with ultramicrosize form.

Preparations: 165 and 330 mg ultra-microsize tablets of Fulvicin P/G; 250 and 500 mg microsize tablets of Fulvicin-U/F; 250 and 500 mg microsize tablets of Grifulvin V; 125, 250, and 500 mg microsize tablets of Grisactin; 125, 200, and 330 mg tablets of Grisactin Ultra (330 mg tablets are scored); 4 oz bottles containing 125 mg/5 mL (1 tsp) of griseofulvin microsize.

Actions: Fungistatic antibiotic; used to treat widespread dermatophyte (fungal) infections.

Clearance: Metabolized via liver.
No change in dosage needed for impaired renal function.

Side Effects: Headache, nausea and vomiting, hypersensitivity reactions, photosensitivity.

Drug Interactions: May need to adjust warfarin dose when taken concomitantly. Barbiturates decrease its activity. Induces increased hepatic metabolism of other hepatically metabolized drugs.

Cautions: Contraindicated in hepatocellular failure.

Pearls: Cost $$$ (300 mg generic ≈$67 wholesale/100 tablets, Grisactin 500 ≈$57 wholesale/60 tablets, Grisactin Ultra 330 mg ≈$88 wholesale/100 tablets).
Warn patients to avoid excessive sunlight (because of possible photosensitivity).
Use with alcohol can cause nausea and vomiting, flushing, and light-headedness.
Periodically monitor CBC, liver function, and renal function during long-term use.
Pregnancy category not established.

GUAIFENESIN expectorant (Robitussin; *see also* the various Robitussin preparations)

Dose: 2 tsp of syrup q4h PO prn.

Preparations: 4 and 8 oz bottles of Robitussin; many other preparations.

Actions: Medication that increases fluid production in the respiratory tract, which may help to liquefy and reduce viscosity of secretions; used to treat persistent cough.

Side Effects: Can cause GI upset and diarrhea at higher doses.

Pearls: Cost $.
  Actual ability to stimulate secretions and clinical efficacy are controversial; several reviews of cold medicines find little evidence to support their routine use.
  Pregnancy category C.

GUANABENZ (Wytensin)

Dose: Initial, 4 mg PO bid; maintenance, 4–16 mg PO bid.

Preparations: 4 and 8 mg tablets.

Actions: Centrally acting agent that stimulates cerebral α_2-receptors, causing decrease in sympathetic outflow from the brain; used to treat hypertension.

Clearance: Metabolized in liver to inactive metabolites.
  No change in dosage needed for impaired renal function.
  Reduce dosage in liver disease.

Side Effects: Drowsiness or sedation (frequent), dizziness, weakness, dry mouth.

Pearls: Cost $$$$ ($\approx$$2/d retail).
  Abrupt discontinuance can cause rebound reaction, including elevated BP, tachycardia, anxiety, and insomnia.
  Warn patients of its sedative effects.
  Pregnancy category C.

GUANETHIDINE (Ismelin)

Dose: 10–50 mg PO qd.

Preparations: 10 and 25 mg tablets.

Actions: Peripheral-acting agent that depletes presynaptic norepinephrine stores and decreases norepinephrine release, diminishing sympathetic output; used to treat hypertension.

Clearance: Metabolized via liver; renal excreted; nonrenal metabolism is increased in renal failure.

Slightly increase dosing interval in ESRD (GFR <10 mL/min); no change needed for milder renal impairment.

Dosage should probably be reduced in liver disease.

Side Effects: Postural hypotension (common), impotence or retrograde ejaculation, diarrhea, nasal stuffiness, weakness, edema, bradycardia, azotemia.

Drug Interactions: Tricyclics reverse its antihypertensive effect. Over-the-counter drugs containing α-agonists (epinephrine, phenylpropanolamine, pseudoephedrine) can decrease its antihypertensive effect. Augments effects of antidiabetic agents.

Cautions: Avoid in heart failure and in patients taking MAOI.

Can worsen or exacerbate asthma.

Can exacerbate peptic ulcer disease (through excess parasympathetic activity).

Contraindicated in patients with known or suspected pheochromocytoma or hypovolemia.

Anesthesia can enhance hypotension and precipitate cardiovascular collapse.

Pearls: Cost $$ (≈$0.70/d retail).

Does not cause depression (because of its poor CNS penetration).

Caution patients about possible postural hypotension.

Pregnancy category C.

Habitrol: see NICOTINE transdermal patch

Halcion: see TRIAZOLAM

Haldol: see HALOPERIDOL

HALOPERIDOL (Haldol)

Dose: Route and disease dependent.
PO: 0.5–5.0 mg bid–tid.
IM: 2–5 mg; may require further IM doses.
"Sundowning": 0.5 mg or more PO or IM q4–6h prn.

Preparations: 1, 2, 5, and 10 mg tablets; 2 mg/mL liquid concentrate; 5 mg/mL injection.

Actions: Butyrophenone that acts as a major tranquilizer and antipsychotic; used to treat significant anxiety, "sundowning" (the phenomenon in which elderly patients become confused at night), and many other psychological conditions.

Clearance: Metabolized via liver; renal excreted.
No change in dosage needed for impaired renal function.
May need to adjust dosage in liver disease (these patients are more sensitive to CNS effects of phenothiazines).
Supplemental dose not required after HD or PD.

Side Effects: Parkinsonian symptoms and other extrapyramidal reactions, tardive dyskinesia, neuroleptic malignant syndrome, confusion and numerous other CNS effects, transient increase or decrease in WBCs, elevated LFTs, dry mouth, blurred vision, urine retention, diaphoresis, priapism, laryngospasm and bronchospasm, numerous GI effects, hyponatremia, increased or decreased glucose level.

Drug Interactions: Can potentiate CNS depressant effects of other CNS depressants. Concomitant use with lithium can increase risk of neuroleptic malignant syndrome.

Cautions: Contraindicated in Parkinson's disease. Use with caution in patients with history of seizures (can lower the seizure threshold), severe cardiac disorders (can cause hypotension or angina), or thyrotoxicosis.

Pearls: Cost: generic $$, Haldol $$$ (100 tablets retail: 5 mg generic ≈$50, 5 mg Haldol ≈$130).

Signs and symptoms of overdose include severe extrapyramidal reactions, hypotension, and oversedation.

Signs of neuroleptic malignant syndrome include extreme rise in temperature, muscle rigidity and "lead-pipe" syndrome, mental status changes, autonomic instability including irregular pulse or BP, greatly increased HR, diaphoresis, arrhythmias, rhabdomyolysis (with increased CPK, myoglobinuria, and acute renal failure).

Pregnancy category C.

HCTZ: see HYDROCHLOROTHIAZIDE

HEPARIN

Dose: Highly variable; often 5000 unit bolus, then 1000 units/h IV.

Some sources are leaning toward a more aggressive initial approach using (either or both) a higher bolus and higher initial infusion rate, such as 1200 units/h IV.

For prophylaxis of deep vein thrombosis, usual dosage is 5000 units SQ q12h.

Actions: Medication that potentiates anticoagulant action of antithrombin III; used to treat unstable angina, venous and arterial thrombosis, and many other clinical conditions.

Clearance: Metabolized via liver; renal excreted; different sources list both increased and decreased $t_{1/2}$ in liver dysfunction.

No change in dosage needed for impaired renal function.

One source that addresses dosage adjustment in liver disease does not recommend any change.

Supplemental dose not required after HD or PD.

Side Effects: Excess bleeding, mild decrease in platelets (common), significant decrease in platelets (rarer), thrombosis, rare hyperkalemia.

Cautions: Contraindicated in patients with active bleeding, severe hypertension, ulcers, hemorrhagic CVA, pericarditis, metastases from hemorrhagic tumors, or recent surgery of the CNS or prostate.

Check with an ophthalmologist before giving to patients with retinopathy.

Use with caution in patients taking platelet-inhibiting drugs.

Pearls: Cost $ (≈$20/d wholesale).

Resistance to its effects is increased in thrombosis, phlebitis, infection, cancer, and postoperatively.

Discontinue if platelets fall <100,000 without other clear cause.

Discontinue if thrombosis (also called "white clot syndrome") develops.

Its role in CVA is controversial (*see "2nd ACCP Conference on Antithrombotic Therapy" in Chest* 95(2):suppl, Feb 1989); a bolus dose is often not given when anticoagulating for CVA (can increase the incidence of CNS hemorrhage).

Pregnancy category C.

Dosage Adjustments:
There are almost as many methods for adjusting IV heparin to PTT levels as there are tired interns. The regimen listed below, used in an Activase protocol, is designed to keep PTT at 1.5–2 times control. It suggests that PTT be monitored regularly and checked 3 h after any dosage change.

PTT	*Adjustment*
3 [x] control	Decrease infusion rate by 50%
2–3 [x] control	Decrease infusion rate by 25%
1.5–2 [x] control	No change
1.5 [x] control	Increase infusion rate by 25% to max of 2500 units/h

Hismanal: see ASTEMIZOLE

HOMATROPINE

Dose: Instill 1 drop (written "gtt") into the eye; may be instilled up to qid in iritis.

Actions: Cycloplegic agent that paralyzes sphincter and ciliary muscles; used to treat iritis.

Pearls: Onset is 30 min; duration of action up to 24 h.

To decrease systemic absorption, compress the lacrimal sac with a finger for 1 min after instilling drops.

Hydeltrasol: see PREDNISOLONE

Hydeltra-T.B.A.: see PREDNISOLONE

HYDRALAZINE (Apresoline)

Dose: Route dependent.

PO: Initial, 10 mg qid for 2–4 days, then 25 mg qid until end of first week, then 50 mg qid.

IV: 20–40 mg IM or IV.

Preparations: 10, 25, 50, and 100 mg tablets; 20 mg/mL injection vials.

Actions: Direct vasodilator; used to treat hypertension.

Clearance: Metabolized via liver; renal excreted.

Slightly increase dosing interval in ESRD; no change needed for milder renal dysfunction.

Supplemental dose not required after HD or PD.

Side Effects: Postural hypotension, headache, GI discomfort, tachycardia, angina, palpitations, peripheral neuritis, SLE-like reaction, (+) Coombs' reaction, blood dyscrasias.

Drug Interactions: Decreases serum levels of propranolol and metoprolol.

Cautions: Contraindicated in CAD and rheumatic mitral valve disease.

Pearls: Cost: generic $, Apresoline $$$ (generic ≈$0.20/d retail, Apresoline ≈$1.80/d retail).

Can cause severe hypotension when given to patients taking diazoxide.

Increases risk of hypotension in patients taking MAOI.

Increases renal blood flow.

Pregnancy category C.

Hydrea: *see* HYDROXYUREA

HYDROCHLOROTHIAZIDE (HCTZ, HydroDIURIL, Thiuretic, etc.; *see also* Aldactazide, Capozide, Dyazide, Maxzide, Moduretic, Prinzide, Zestoretic)

Dose: 25–100 mg PO qod–qd.

Preparations: 25, 50, and 100 mg tablets; also available for certain brands as 50 mg/5 mL (1 tsp) oral solution.

Actions: Thiazide diuretic; used to treat hypertension and edema.

Clearance: Renal excreted.
Avoid in ESRD.
No change in dosage needed for liver disease.

Side Effects: Hypokalemia, hypomagnesemia, dilutional hyponatremia, orthostatic hypotension, glycosuria, hyperuricemia, GI discomfort, pancreatitis.

Drug Interactions: Cholestyramine and cholestipol reduce its absorption.

Cautions: Use with caution, if at all, in patients with history of glucose intolerance, gout, or sulfa allergy.

Pearls: Cost $ (100 tablets retail: 50 mg generic $\approx$\$5, 50 mg HydroDIURIL $\approx$\$17).
Follow serum K^+.
Can detrimentally alter lipid and glucose metabolism.
25 mg dose is as effective as higher doses in treatment of hypertension.
Pregnancy category B.

HYDROCODONE: *see* Vicodin, Vicodin ES

HYDROCORTISONE (Hydrocortone, Solu-Cortef; *see also* HYDROCORTISONE suppositories, HYDROCORTISONE topical cream)

Dose: Preparation and route dependent.

Hydrocortone (hydrocortisone sodium phosphate): PO, 20–240 mg qd; IM or IV, 7.5–120 mg q12h.

Solu-Cortef (hydrocortisone sodium succinate): IM or IV, 100–500 mg q2–10h prn.

Preparations: 10 and 20 mg tablets of Hydrocortone; 2 and 10 mL vials containing 50 mg/mL of Hydrocortone; 100, 250, 500, and 1000 mg powder-containing vials of Solu-Cortef.

Actions: Corticosteroid; used to treat adrenocortical insufficiency (one of two drugs of choice). May also be used intra-articularly and topically.

Clearance: Metabolized via liver.

No change in dosage needed for impaired renal function.

Dosage adjustment probably not needed for liver disease.

Side Effects (acute): Na^+ and water retention (leading to increases in hypertension, edema, and CHF), elevated glucose, psychiatric disturbances ("steroid psychosis"), impaired wound healing, increased risk of peptic ulcer disease, increased catabolism.

Side Effects (chronic): Myopathy, osteoporosis, vertebral compression fractures, aseptic necrosis, CNS changes, edema.

Drug Interactions: Decreases hypoglycemic effects of insulin and OHAs. Concomitant use with K^+-depleting diuretics increases risk of hypokalemia. Prolongs or shortens PT in patients taking warfarin. Phenytoin, phenobarbital, and rifampin increase its clearance and reduce its serum level.

Pearls: Cost $$ (20 mg Hydrocortone $31 wholesale/100 tablets).

Can mask signs of infection.

Patients may need "stress-dose" steroids during stress; usual stress dose for severe illness or surgery, 100 mg IV q8h.

Pregnancy category not established.

Relative steroid activity:

	Relative anti-inflammatory and glucocorticoid activity	*Relative mineralocorticoid activity*
hydrocortisone	1.0	1.0
prednisone	4.0	0.8
methylprednisolone	5.0	0.5
dexamethasone	25–30	0.0

HYDROCORTISONE suppositories (Anusol-HC, other brands)

Dose: 1 suppository PR bid–tid.

Preparations: 25 mg suppositories of Anusol-HC.

Actions: Topical corticosteroid containing hydrocortisone; used to treat hemorrhoids.

Side Effects: Local irritation and reactions. Can theoretically suppress adrenocortical axis if enough is absorbed.

Pearls: Cost $$$ (Anusol-HC suppository ≈$2 retail).
Pregnancy category C.

HYDROCORTISONE topical cream (Anusol-HC and many other brands)

Dose: Apply to skin bid–qid.

Preparations: 0.25%, 0.5%, and 1.0% are usual concentrations; Anusol-HC available only as 2.5% preparation in 30 g tube.

Actions: Weak topical steroid; used to treat many dermatologic conditions.

Side Effects: Local irritation and reactions. Can theoretically suppress adrenocortical axis if enough is absorbed.

Pearls: Cost $ (tube ≈$5 retail).
Pregnancy category C.

Hydrocortone: *see* **HYDROCORTISONE**

HydroDIURIL: *see* **HYDROCHLOROTHIAZIDE**

HYDROMORPHONE (Dilaudid)

Dose: Route dependent.
  PO: 2–4 mg q4–6h prn.
  SQ or IM: Suggested starting dose, 1–2 mg q4–6h prn.
  Suppository: 3 mg q4–6h prn.

Preparations: 1, 2, 3, and 4 mg tablets; 3 mg suppositories; 1, 2, 3, 4, and 10 mg/mL injection.

Actions: Narcotic analgesic; used to treat moderate to severe pain.

Clearance: Little information available; probably metabolized via liver.
  One source recommends using with caution in hepatic or renal failure.

Side Effects: Drowsiness, mood changes, mental clouding, depressed respiratory drive and cough, nausea and vomiting, pinpoint pupils, increased parasympathetic activity, elevated CSF pressure, decreased BP, dizziness, agitation.

Cautions: Contraindicated in patients with CNS injury or lesions.
  Use with caution in elderly or debilitated patients and in patients with impaired hepatic or renal function, hypothyroidism, Addison's disease, prostate hypertrophy, or urethral stricture.

Pearls: Cost $$$ (100 tablets retail: 2 mg generic ≈$33, 2 mg Dilaudid ≈$43).
  Pregnancy category C.

HYDROXOCOBALAMIN: *see* COBALAMIN

HYDROXYUREA (Hydrea)

Dose: Tumor dependent. Usually given qd or q3d. Can only be given PO.

Preparations: 500 mg tablets.

Actions: Antineoplastic agent that probably inhibits DNA synthesis; used to treat myeloproliferative disorders.

Clearance: Predominantly renal excreted.
Moderately to markedly reduced dosage in impaired renal function.

Side Effects: Bone marrow suppression, stomatitis, anorexia, nausea and vomiting, diarrhea and constipation, megaloblastic erythropoiesis (not related to vitamin B_{12} or folate deficiency), occasional impairment of renal tubular function or alopecia.

Cautions: Contraindicated if WBCs <2500 or platelets <100,000.
Relatively contraindicated during pregnancy.

Pearls: Cost $$$ ($121 wholesale/100 tablets).
Follow CBC, LFTs, BUN, and creatinine.
Bone marrow suppression is dose-limiting side effect.
During pregnancy, known teratogenic potential must be weighed against potential benefits.

HYDROXYZINE (Atarax, Vistaril)

Dose: Disease dependent.
Anxiety: 50–100 mg PO qid.
Pruritus: 25 mg PO tid–qid.
Nausea and vomiting: 25–50 mg IM.
Sedation before and after anesthesia: 50–100 mg PO or 25–100 mg IM.

Preparations: Atarax: available as 10, 25, 50, and 100 mg tablets and as syrup containing 10 mg/5 mL (1 tsp); Vistaril: available as 25, 50, and 100 mg capsules and in vials for IM injection.

Actions: Drug chemically unrelated to either phenothiazines or benzodiazepines, with anxiolytic, antipruritic, and antihistamine properties; used to treat anxiety, nausea and vomiting, as a sedative, and as an antipruritic.

Clearance: Little data available for humans; undergoes extensive hepatic metabolism in rats.

Side Effects: Dry mouth, drowsiness, rare tremor and convulsions.

Cautions: Should not be used during early pregnancy or in potentially pregnant patients.

Pearls: Cost: generic $$, Vistaril $$$$ (100 tablets retail: 50 mg generic ≈$12–$20, 50 mg Vistaril ≈$80–$100).
Potentiates CNS depressant effects of other CNS depressants.
Contraindicated in early pregnancy.

Hytrin: *see* **TERAZOSIN**

IBUPROFEN (Advil, Medipren, Motrin, Motrin IB, Nuprin, Rufen)

Dose: 200–800 mg PO qid.

Preparations: 300, 400, 600, and 800 mg tablets of Motrin; 200 mg tablets of Advil, Medipren, Motrin IB, and Nuprin.

Actions: NSAID with analgesic and antipyretic activity that may work by inhibiting prostaglandin synthetase; used to treat inflammatory conditions and for pain relief.

Clearance: Metabolized via liver.
No change in dosage needed for impaired renal function.

Side Effects: GI bleeding and ulceration, fluid retention and edema, elevated LFTs, interstitial nephritis and exacerbation of "prerenal" renal failure, rash, prolonged bleeding time (from reversible platelet inhibition), dizziness, visual changes.

Drug Interactions: Reduces renal clearance of methotrexate. Decreases natriuretic effect of diuretics. Raises serum level of lithium.

Cautions: Use with *extreme* caution, if at all, in patients with history of upper GI bleeding or ulcer and in elderly patients.
Should not be used by women who wish to become pregnant (can cause uterine muscle contraction).
Can cause premature closure of ductus arteriosus or complications during delivery when used during last trimester of pregnancy.

Pearls: Cost $$ (100 tablets retail: 200 mg generic ≈$5, 600 mg generic ≈$16, 600 mg Motrin ≈$20); at ≈$1/d, Motrin is about half the cost of most other NSAIDs.

200 mg preparation is available over-the-counter without a prescription.

Consider use of misoprostol (Cytotec) to protect the stomach during long-term therapy in patients at increased risk of upper GI bleeding.

Should not be used during third trimester of pregnancy.

IL-2: see INTERLEUKIN-2

IFEX: see IFOSFAMIDE

IFOSFAMIDE (IFEX)

Dose: 1.2 g/m^2 IV daily for 5 consecutive days; repeat q3wk or after recovery from hematologic toxicity.

Actions: Antineoplastic alkylating agent, chemically related to nitrogen mustard and a synthetic analog of cyclophosphamide, that cross-links tumor cell DNA; used to treat malignancies.

Clearance: Hydroxylated to active metabolite by liver enzymes; activation of the inactive drug to its active metabolite may theoretically be less in patients with liver disease.

Use with caution in impaired renal function.

Side Effects: Hemorrhagic cystitis, myelosuppression, alopecia, nausea and vomiting, CNS toxicity (somnolence, confusion, depressive psychosis, hallucinations), renal toxicity (usually tubular damage).

Drug Interactions Concomitant use with other chemotherapeutic agents increases myelosuppression.

Cautions: Contraindicated in patients with severely depressed bone marrow or significant microscopic hematuria.

Pearls: To decrease the incidence of hemorrhagic cystitis, give with an agent such as mesna and hydrate vigorously.

If microscopic hematuria (>10 RBCs/high power field) is present, withhold subsequent doses until resolved. Check urinalysis periodically after treatment.

Obtain CBC prior to use and periodically after treatment; postpone treatment for WBCs <2000 or platelets <50,000.

Pregnancy category D.

Ilotycin: see ERYTHROMYCIN ophthalmic ointment

IMIPENEM: see Primaxin

Imodium: see LOPERAMIDE

Imuran: see AZATHIOPRINE

INDAPAMIDE (Lozol)

Dose: 2.5 mg PO qd.

Preparations: 2.5 mg tablets.

Actions: Diuretic with some additional vasodilating actions; used to treat hypertension and CHF.

Side Effects: Headache, dizziness, fatigue, anxiety or irritability, muscle cramps, numbness of extremities, hypokalemia.

Drug Interactions: Manufacturer notes that diuretics generally should not be used concomitantly with lithium (they reduce its renal clearance and add to risk of lithium toxicity).

Pearls: Cost $$$ ($\approx$$20/mo retail).

Manufacturer notes that doses of 5.0 mg or higher are associated with more frequent and severe hypokalemia with no apparent additional benefit in the treatment of hypertension or CHF.

Its advantages over hydrochlorothiazide include less K^+ wasting, less elevation of uric acid levels, and fewer adverse effects on lipid profiles and glucose tolerance.

Pregnancy category B.

Inderal, Inderal LA: see PROPRANOLOL

Indocin, Indocin SR: see INDOMETHACIN

INDOMETHACIN (Indocin, Indocin SR)

Dose: Preparation dependent.
Indocin: 25–50 mg PO tid (with food or antacids) or one 50 mg rectal suppository bid–tid.
Indocin SR: One 75 mg capsule PO qd–bid.

Preparations: Indocin: 25 and 50 mg capsules; 237 mL bottle of oral suspension containing 25 mg/5 mL (1 tsp); 50 mg rectal suppositories. Indocin SR: 75 mg sustained-release capsules.

Actions: Nonsteroidal anti-inflammatory agent with analgesic and antipyretic actions; used to treat inflammation and for pain relief.

Clearance: Metabolized via liver.
Sources disagree on whether dosage should be changed in impaired renal function.
Supplemental dose not required after HD.

Side Effects: GI irritation, nausea, dyspepsia, upper GI bleeding, proteinuria, interstitial nephritis, nephrotic syndrome, worsening of "prerenal" renal failure, prolonged bleeding time, CNS effects (especially in elderly patients).

Cautions: Contraindicated in patients with salicylate sensitivity, ulcer, or history of upper GI bleeding.
Can cause premature closure of the ductus arteriosus when used during last trimester of pregnancy.

Pearls: Cost: generic $$, Indocin $$$ (100 tablets retail: 50 mg generic ≈$27, 50 mg Indocin ≈$80); Motrin is similar in cost to generic indomethacin and less than half the daily cost of Indocin.
Should not be used during third trimester of pregnancy.

Inflamase, Inflamase Forte: see PREDNISOLONE SODIUM PHOSPHATE eye drops

INH: see ISONIAZID

Inocor: see AMRINONE

INSULIN

Dose: Highly variable. One suggested initial dose is 10–20 mg NPH or Humulin N SQ every morning with dosage adjustments based on subsequent fingerstick glucose tests.

Preparations: *See under* Pearls.

Clearance: Metabolized via liver; renal excreted.
Slight reduction in dosage in impaired renal function is generally suggested.
Special care should be taken when adjusting dosage in patients with worsening renal failure (the body's needs for insulin can sometimes rise or fall).

Side Effects: Local reactions, severe systemic allergic reactions, insulin reaction (symptoms include fatigue, nervousness, confusion, trembling, headache, nausea, cold sweats), hunger, weight gain.

Drug Interactions: Concomitant use of alcohol, disopyramide, MAOI, OHA, or high-dose salicylates increases risk of hypoglycemia. Concomitant use with steroids, diuretics, phenytoin, sympathomimetics, or thyroid hormone increases risk of hyperglycemia.

Pearls: Cost $$ (10 mL bottle containing 100 units/mL: regular, Lente, NPH, PZI, Ultralente beef insulin ≈$12 retail; Humulin R, Humulin N, Humulin L, Humulin U recombinant insulin ≈$14 retail); cost differential between beef insulin and human insulin manufactured through recombinant DNA is surprisingly little.
Insulin requirements are increased in high fever, obesity, hyperthyroidism, severe infection, trauma, surgery, and Cushing's syndrome.
Insulin requirements may be decreased in hepatic dysfunction, impaired renal function, hypothyroidism, nausea and vomiting, increased activity (exercise), hypopituitarism, and adrenal insufficiency.
Only regular insulin can be given IV.
Does not cross the placenta, and benefits of treatment probably outweigh any potential risks during pregnancy.

"Sliding-Scale" Insulin Protocol:

While in the hospital, many patients are put on a "sliding-scale" regimen of regular short-acting insulin, given SQ q4h or q6h, with the dose based on fingerstick glucose levels. When such a regimen is ordered, dosage should be based on the patient's usual insulin requirements. Patients should rarely receive morning doses of longer-acting insulin while on a sliding-scale insulin regimen (both can peak at the same time and cause hypoglycemia: NPH given at 7 AM and regular insulin given at 11 AM would both peak at 3 PM). A "typical" regimen follows, though all physicians and diabetologists have their own approach:

Regular insulin SQ, sliding scale q6h, with fingerstick glucose tests:

Glucose level of 0–180:	0 units
181–240:	2 units
241–300:	3 units
301–350:	4 units
351–400:	5 units
>400:	call M.D.

Available mixtures and kinetics:

	Onset	Peak	Duration
Regular insulin (regular insulin, Humulin R)	1/2–1 h	2–4 h	5–7 h
Prompt insulin zinc suspension (Semilente)	1–3 h	2–8 h	12–16 h
Isophane insulin suspension (NPH, Humulin N)	3–4 h	6–12 h	24–48 h
Insulin zinc suspension (Lente, Humulin L)	1–3 h	8–12 h	24–48 h
Protamine zinc insulin (PZI)	4–6 h	14–24 h	36 h
Extended insulin zinc suspension (Ultralente, Humulin U)	4–6 h	18–24 h	36 h

Intal: see CROMOLYN SODIUM

Intropin: *see* **DOPAMINE**

INTERFERON (ALPHA INTERFERON, Intron A, Roferon-A)

Dose: Dose dependent; given IM or SQ.

Actions: Naturally occurring single-chain proteins that bind to specific cell membrane receptors. Their numerous effects include enhancing synthesis of antiviral enzymes, enhancing cellular antigen expression, increasing activity of natural killer cells and phagocytic macrophages, and antitumor actions.

Clearance: Sources vary. *PDR* states that interferons are filtered in the glomeruli and undergo proteolytic degradation during tubular reabsorption; another source notes that the majority of a dose is thought to be metabolized with none filtered or secreted by the kidneys.

Side Effects: Numerous, some quite common: extremely frequent flulike symptoms (including fever, fatigue, myalgia, headache, chills, arthralgias), extremely frequent GI symptoms (including anorexia, nausea and vomiting, diarrhea, abdominal pain), extremely frequent dizziness, cough, alopecia, weight loss, dryness or inflammation of the oropharynx, rash, night sweats, pruritus, change in taste, confusion and mental status changes, paresthesias and numbness, elevated LFTs, leukopenia, neutropenia, thrombocytopenia.

Cautions: Use with caution in patients with severe cardiac disease, renal disease, hepatic disease, seizure disorders, or CNS dysfunction.

Pearls: Cost $$$1/2 ($40 wholesale/5 million units).
Pregnancy category C.

INTERLEUKIN-2 (IL-2, Proleukin)

Dose: Disease and regimen dependent; given IV.

Actions: Lymphokine protein that binds to T cells and, among its actions, induces mitosis and cell transformation, stimulates helper

T cells, and induces production of cytotoxic lymphocytes with antitumor activity; used to treat malignancies.

Clearance: Believed to be primarily renal metabolized.

Side Effects: Fever and chills, nausea and vomiting, rash and pruritus, nasal congestion, fluid retention and pulmonary edema, hypotension.

Drug Interactions: Glucocorticoids block all its actions.

Cautions: Use with caution in patients with history of cardiopulmonary disease.

Pearls: Its hypotensive effects usually occur 2–4 h after injection.
  Follow BP and fluid status and periodically examine the lungs for signs of pulmonary edema.

Intron A: see INTERFERON

Intropin: see DOPAMINE

IODINATED GYCEROL: see Organidin

IPECAC syrup

Dose: 15–30 mL of syrup with 200–300 mL water.

Preparations: Solution containing 70 mg/mL.

Actions: Emetic that induces vomiting; used to treat recent drug overdose.

Side Effects: Cardiovascular disturbances if absorbed (which can occur if not vomited within 30 min of ingestion or if chronically abused).

Drug Interactions: Activated charcoal neutralizes its emetic effect.

Cautions: Contraindicated in patients who have ingested caustic substances or petroleum distillates. Use with caution in esophageal disease.

Pearls: Induces vomiting within 30 min in >90% of patients. Average onset of action <20 min.

IPRATROPIUM (Atrovent)

Dose: Usual, 2 inhalations from metered-dose inhaler qid; max, 12 inhalations in 24 h.

Preparations: 14 g metered-dose inhaler, supplied with mouthpiece, that provides sufficient medicine for 200 inhalations.

Actions: Anticholinergic bronchodilator, chemically related to atropine, that blocks smooth muscle muscarinic receptors; used to treat reactive airway disease.

Side Effects: Cough, dry mouth, bad taste, palpitations, nervousness, paradoxical decline in pulmonary function tests with bronchoconstriction, dizziness, headache, GI distress.

Cautions: Use with caution in narrow-angle glaucoma, prostate hypertrophy, or bladder neck obstruction.

Pearls: Cost $$$ (inhaler ≈$30 retail).
Pregnancy category B.

IRON: see FERROUS SULFATE

Ismelin: see GUANETHIDINE

ISOETHARINE (Bronkometer, Bronkosol)

Dose: Delivery dependent.
Bronkometer: 1 or 2 inhalations, usually no more frequently than q4h.
Bronkosol nebulizer: 0.5 mL in 2.5 mL NS q2–4h.

Preparations: Bronkometer: available in 10 and 15 mL vials with oral nebulizer.

Actions: Sympathomimetic amine with β_2 affinity that produces bronchodilatation; used to treat reactive airway disease.

Side Effects: Headache, anxiety, restlessness, tremor, insomnia, dizziness, tachycardia, palpitations, BP changes, nausea.

Cautions: Use with caution in patients with CAD, arrhythmias, hypertension, or hyperthyroidism.

Pearls: Cost $$$ (retail cost of inhaler: Bronkometer ≈$20–$28, Bronkosol ≈$16–$20).
Pregnancy category not established.

ISONIAZID (INH, Nydrazid)

Dose: 300 mg PO qd.

Preparations: 50, 100, and 300 mg tablets; 50 mg/5 mL (1 tsp) syrup.

Actions: Antimycobacterial antibiotic that inhibits synthesis of mycolic acid; used to treat mycobacterial infections.

Clearance: Metabolized primarily via liver; 5–30% excreted unchanged in urine.
Slightly decrease dosage for slow acetylators with impaired renal function.
Reduce dosage in moderate to severe liver disease.
Supplemental dose suggested after HD or PD.

Side Effects: Elevated LFTs and hepatitis (age related), peripheral neuropathy (especially in diabetics, alcohol abusers, and malnourished patients), pyridoxine (vitamin B_6) deficiency, reduced WBCs, mental status changes, (+) ANA titer.

Drug Interactions: Reduces excretion of phenytoin or enhances its effects.

Cautions: Contraindicated in active liver disease. Try to avoid in pregnant or potentially pregnant patients.

Pearls: Cost $ (≈$14 retail/100 tablets).
Often given with pyridoxine 10 mg PO qd to prevent peripheral neuritis.
Follow LFTs.
Pregnancy category not established and available data conflicting; consider beginning preventive therapy *after* delivery if possible.

Isoptin, Isoptin SR: see VERAPAMIL

Isopto Atropine: see ATROPINE eye drops

Isopto Carpine see PILOCARPINE

Isopto Hyoscine: see SCOPOLAMINE eye drops

Isordil, Isordil Tembids: see ISOSORBIDE DINITRATE

ISOSORBIDE DINITRATE (Isordil, Isordil Tembids)

Dose: Preparation dependent.
  Regular-acting: 10–40 mg PO qid.
  Long-acting: 40–80 mg PO bid–tid of Isordil Tembids.

Preparations: 5, 10, 20, 30, and 40 mg tablets; 40 mg long-acting Isordil Tembids.

Actions: Vasodilator (mainly of veins and coronary arteries); used to treat CAD.

Clearance: Metabolized via liver; 20% renal excreted.
  No change in dosage needed for impaired renal function.

Side Effects: Hypotension, reflex tachycardia, headache and flushing.
  Can cause anemia in patients with GGPD deficiency.

Pearls: Cost $ (≈$10 retail/100 tablets).
  A drug-free interval is recommended to avoid developing tolerance.
  Pregnancy category C.

ISOTRETINOIN (Accutane)

Dose: 0.25–1.0 mg/kg PO bid.

Preparations: 10, 20, and 40 mg capsules.

Actions: Retinoid that inhibits sebaceous gland function and keratinization; used to treat recalcitrant cystic acne.

Side Effects: Dry skin, skin fragility, pruritus, epistaxis, dry nose and mouth, cheilitis, conjunctivitis, skeletal hyperostosis, arthralgias and other musculoskeletal symptoms, elevated LFTs and CPK, proteinuria, hematuria, increased triglycerides, worsening of serum glucose levels, reduced tolerance for contact lenses, pseudotumor cerebri. (*All these side effects are relatively common!*) Also associated with many less common side effects and reactions.

Cautions: Contraindicated in pregnant or potentially pregnant patients.

Pearls: Cost $ (≈$3 retail/100 tablets).
Patients should not take multivitamin preparations containing vitamin A (to avoid possible toxicity).
Follow LFTs, triglycerides, and serum glucose.
Warn patients of possible reduced tolerance for contact lenses, of the absolute necessity to avoid pregnancy, of frequent side effects listed above, and to avoid donating blood during therapy and for at least 1 month afterward.
Pregnancy category X: has been associated with *major* fetal abnormalities.

ISRADIPINE (DynaCirc)

Dose: Initial, 2.5 mg PO bid; maintenance, 2.5–10 mg PO bid.

Preparations: 2.5 and 5 mg capsules.

Actions: Calcium-channel blocker; used to treat hypertension.

Clearance: Metabolized primarily via liver.
May need to reduce dosage in liver and renal disease (because bioavailability is increased), but starting dose should remain unchanged.

Side Effects: Dizziness, edema, tachycardia, palpitations, flushing.

Pearls: Cost $$$ (≈$1.40/d retail).
Allow 2–4 weeks to achieve maximum antihypertensive effect before adjusting dosage.
Pregnancy category C.

Kabikinase: *see* **STREPTOKINASE**

KAOLIN: *see* **Kaopectate liquid**

Kaopectate liquid (KAOLIN + PECTIN)

Dose: 60–120 mL (4–8 Tbsp) PO after each bowel movement or prn.

Preparations: 3, 8, 12, and 16 oz and 1 gallon bottles.

Pearls: Cost $.
  Can reduce absorption of other PO drugs.
  Pregnancy category C.

Kaopectate tablets (300 mg ATTAPULGITE)

Dose: 1200 mg (4 tablets) PO after each bowel movement; max, 14 tablets in 24 h. Swallow tablets whole with water.

Preparations: Packs of 16 tablets.

Kayexalate: *see* **SODIUM POLYSTYRENE SULFONATE**

K-Dur: *see* **POTASSIUM CHLORIDE**

K-Phos: *see* **PHOSPHORUS**

Keflex: *see* **CEPHALEXIN**

Keftab: *see* **CEPHALEXIN**

Kefurox *see* **CEFUROXIME**

Kefzol: *see* **CEFAZOLIN**

Kenalog: *see* **TRIAMCINOLONE ACETONIDE cream, lotion, and ointment**

KETOCONAZOLE (Nizoral)

Dose: Usual lower dose, 200 mg PO qd; maximum dose varies from 600–1200 mg daily with different sources.

When used to treat resistant fungal infections of the skin, use low doses (such as 200 mg PO qd).

May be taken without regard to meals.

Preparations: 200 mg tablets.

Actions: Synthetic agent that impairs synthesis of ergosterol (a vital component of fungal cell membranes); used to treat fungal infections.

Clearance: Metabolized via liver; biliary excreted.

No change in dosage needed for impaired renal function.

Reduce dosage, if used at all, in significant liver disease.

Side Effects: Nausea and vomiting, elevated LFTs and hepatotoxicity, rash, pruritus, adrenal suppression, gynecomastia, blood dyscrasias.

Drug Interactions: Antacids, sucralfate, H_2 blockers, and omeprazole decrease its absorption (requires acidity for dissolution). Isoniazid and rifampin reduce its serum level. Raises serum level of cyclosporin A. Can prolong PT in patients taking warfarin. Coadministration with phenytoin can alter metabolism of both drugs.

Pearls: Cost $$$ (≈$35 retail/2 wk of therapy).

No significant CSF penetration.

Check LFTs before and at frequent intervals during therapy.

Pregnancy category C.

KETOCONAZOLE topical (Nizoral topical)

Dose: Apply to skin qd–bid.

Preparations: 15 and 60 g tubes of 2% cream.

Actions: Topical antifungal; used to treat tinea infections.

Side Effects: Skin irritation, stinging, pruritus, allergic reactions.

Pearls: Cost $$$$ (60 g tube ≈$41 retail).

Pregnancy category C.

KETOROLAC (Toradol)

Dose: 30–60 mg IM loading dose, then 15–30 mg IM q6h.

Actions: NSAID that may be given IM for short-term management of pain.

Clearance: $t_{1/2}$ is prolonged in renal failure and in elderly patients.

Reduce dosage in renal failure, in elderly patients, and in patients weighing <50 kg.

Side Effects: GI distress, drowsiness, worsening of "prerenal" renal failure. Chronic use can cause kidney damage.

Cautions: Contraindicated in patients with allergy to ASA or NSAID, nasal polyps, or history of angioedema.

Use with extreme caution in patients with CHF, ascites, cirrhosis, or decreased renal function, and in elderly patients.

Pearls: Cost $$ (30 mg ≈$30 wholesale).

Onset of action is 10–15 min; peak effect occurs within 2 h.

Can have comparable analgesic effect to meperidine and morphine.

Pregnancy category B.

Klonopin: see CLONAZEPAM

Kwell: see LINDANE cream and lotion

LABETOLOL (Normodyne, Trandate)

Dose: Delivery dependent.

PO: Initial, 100 mg bid; may be increased q2–3d in increments of 100 mg bid. Usual maintenance, 200–400 mg bid; max, 600–1200 mg bid.

IV: Initial, 20 mg IV over 2 min; additional doses of 40–80 mg may be given at 10-min intervals until satisfactory response or total of 300 mg is reached.

Preparations: 100, 200, and 300 mg tablets; vials of 5 mg/mL for injection.

Actions: Nonselective β-blocker that also selectively blocks α₁-receptors; used to treat hypertension.

Clearance: Metabolized primarily via liver.
No change in dosage needed for impaired renal function.
Reduce dosage in liver disease.
Supplemental dose not required after HD or PD.

Side Effects: Fatigue, dizziness, nausea, worsening of heart failure, bronchospasm, rare liver toxicity.

Drug Interactions: Cimetidine increases its bioavailability.

Cautions: Contraindicated in CHF, reactive airway disease, severe bradycardia, and second- or third-degree heart block.

Pearls: Maximum effect of IV dose usually occurs within 5 min after injection.
Does not lead to significant bradycardia.
When discontinuing, taper gradually to avoid "β-blocker withdrawal."
Can produce falsely elevated measured levels of urinary catecholamines and false (+) urine tests for amphetamines.
Pregnancy category C.

Lactinex: *see* LACTOBACILLUS

LACTOBACILLUS (Bacid, Lactinex)

Dose: Brand dependent.
Bacid: 2 capsules PO bid–qid with milk.
Lactinex: 1 packet PO tid–qid with food, juice, or milk.

Actions: Preparation used to restore normal intestinal flora after treatment with broad-spectrum antibiotics.

Pearls: Cost $.
Actual clinical efficacy is controversial.
Avoid in fever.
Pregnancy category C.

LACTULOSE

Dose: Disease dependent.
   Laxative: Initial, 15–30 mL PO qd; may increase to 60 mL PO qd.
   Encephalopathy: PO, initially 30–45 mL hourly until diarrhea occurs, then 30–45 mL tid–qid to produce 2 or 3 soft stools each day; PR, 300 mL lactulose with 700 mL water q4–6h.

Preparations: 10 g/15 mL syrup.

Actions: Disaccharide sugar metabolized in the colon to low-molecular-weight acid metabolites that raise osmotic pressure and promote bowel evacuation; also acidifies stool, inhibiting bacterial production of NH_3; used as a laxative and to treat hepatic encephalopathy.

Clearance: >97% not absorbed.

Side Effects: Severe diarrhea, hypernatremia.

Drug Interactions: Concomitant use with neomycin can reduce its effectiveness (can destroy saccharolytic bacteria in the colon).

Pearls: Cost $ (≈$12/d wholesale).
   Pregnancy category B.

Lanoxin: see DIGOXIN

Lasix: see FUROSEMIDE

Leukeran: see CHLORAMBUCIL

Leukine: see GRANULOCYTE-MACROPHAGE COLONY-STIMULATING FACTOR

Levlen oral contraceptive (LEVONORGESTREL + ETHINYL ESTRADIOL)

Dose: 1 tablet PO qd; with 21-day regimen, take no pills on d 22–28 then begin a new cycle (3 weeks on, 1 week off).
   Take first pill of Levlen 21 on day 5 of menstrual cycle.

Take first pill of Levlen 28 the first Sunday after onset of menses, or that Sunday if it is the first day of menses.

Preparations: Available in 21- and 28-pill preparations. Last 7 pills in the 28-pill regimen contain only inert ingredients; active pills contain 0.15 mg levonorgestrel and 0.030 mg ethinyl estradiol.

Actions: Combination oral contraceptive that suppresses ovulation and causes cervical and endometrial changes; used to prevent pregnancy.

Side Effects: Serious vascular complications, menstrual changes, cervical changes, breast changes, vaginal candidiasis, hypertension, edema, weight changes, gallbladder disease, GI distress, nausea and vomiting, liver tumors, migraine headache, rash, depression, glucose intolerance, visual changes from alteration in corneal curvature, intolerance for contact lenses.

Drug Interactions: Contraceptive effectiveness can be decreased by antibiotics (ampicillin, chloramphenicol, isoniazid, nitrofurantoin, penicillin V, phenytoin, rifampin, sulfonamides, tetracycline), analgesics, anxiolytics, antihistamines, migraine preparations, phenylbutazone, phenytoin, and tranquilizers.

Cautions: Contraindicated in thromboembolic or thrombophlebitic disorders, cardiovascular or cerebrovascular disease, genital bleeding of unknown cause, endometrial or other estrogen-dependent tumors, and possible pregnancy.

Cigarette smoking increases risk of serious cardiovascular complications; patients should be *strongly* advised not to smoke.

Pearls: Cost $$$ ($\approx$$20/mo retail); all contraceptive pills are similarly priced.

Patients should undergo complete workup prior to use with special attention to history of abnormal vaginal bleeding, BP, breast examination, and pelvic examination including cervical cytology.

Pregnancy category X.

LEVOBUNOLOL (Betagan)

Dose: Instill 1 or 2 drops (written "gtt") into the eye daily.

Actions: Nonselective β-blocker that decreases production of aqueous humor; used to treat glaucoma.

Side Effects (systemic): Presumably can cause bradycardia, conduction abnormalities, and exacerbation of COPD and asthma.

LEVODOPA: *see* Sinemet

LEVONORGESTREL (Norplant; *see also* Levlen, Tri-Levlen, Triphasil)

Dose: Insert 6 tubes under skin of upper arm.

Preparations: 6 Silastic tubes each containing 36 mg levonorgestrel.

Actions: Contraceptive that inhibits ovulation and thickens cervical mucus; used to prevent pregnancy.

Side Effects: Menstrual changes, increased number of days of bleeding and spotting, headache, depression, nervousness, breast discharge and pain, dizziness, acne, hirsuitism, hair loss, weight gain, local reactions.

Drug Interactions: Phenytoin and carbamazepine can decrease its efficacy.

Cautions: Contraindicated in pregnant or potentially pregnant patients.

Pearls: Cost $$$$ ($350 wholesale).
Pregnancy category X.

Levophed: *see* NOREPINEPHRINE

LEVOTHYROXINE: *see* L-THYROXINE

Levoxine: *see* L-THYROXINE

Librium: *see* CHLORDIAZEPOXIDE

Lidex: see FLUOCINONIDE cream, gel, ointment, and solution

LIDOCAINE (Xylocaine)

Dose: Suggested starting regimens vary slightly. Possible regimens for acute therapy and prophylaxis are as follows.

Acute therapy: 1 mg/kg IV bolus initially; may then give IV bolus of 0.5 mg/kg q5–8min to total loading dose of 3 mg/kg. Begin IV infusion at 1–4 mg/kg/min if therapy is successful (many physicians will start at 2 mg/kg/min).

Prophylaxis: 1 mg/kg loading dose (some physicians will give a second loading bolus of 0.5 mg/kg 15 min after first dose because lidocaine is distributed thoughout the body). Begin IV infusion at 1–4 mg/kg/min after first loading dose (many physicians will start at 2 mg/kg/min).

Actions: Type Ib antiarrhythmic; used to treat ventricular arrhythmias.

Clearance: Metabolized via liver; 20% renal excreted; metabolism is reduced in liver dysfunction, CHF, and shock (because of decreased liver blood flow).

No change in dosage needed for impaired renal function.

In liver disease, give no more than 2 mg/min and follow serum levels.

Reduce dosage in elderly patients, who are more susceptible to lidocaine toxicity.

Supplemental dose not required after HD.

Side Effects: Sedation, irritability, seizures, coma, mental status changes (often referred to as "lidocaine toxicity" and particularly common in elderly patients), respiratory depression, hypotension.

Drug Interactions: Cimetidine decreases its metabolism. β-blockers can reduce its clearance (by decreasing liver blood flow).

Pearls: Cost $ (≈$2/d wholesale).

May give 300 mg IM if no IV access is available.

Give with caution: onset of action is 5 to 15 min.

In acute myocardial infarction, prophylactic may increase the incidence of ventricular ectopy, but has not been shown to have any effect on mortality. Concerns about the increased incidence of asystole lidocaine.

Pregnancy category B.

LINDANE cream and lotion (Kwell)

Dose: Disease dependent.
Scabies: Apply thin layer and massage in; wash off after 8–12 h.
Lice: Apply and work into hair; add water after 4 min, then rinse and towel.

Preparations: 2 oz cream; 2 oz, 1 pint, and 1 gallon lotion; 2 oz, 1 pint, and 1 gallon shampoo.

Actions: Topical antiparasitic agent; used to treat lice and scabies.

Side Effects: Skin irritation, pruritus. Excessive absorption can lead to CNS effects ranging from dizziness to convulsion.

Cautions: Contraindicated in patients with known seizure disorders.

Pearls: Cost: generic $$, Kwell $$$$ (1 pint generic ≈$25 retail, 1 pint Kwell ≈$65 retail).
Pregnancy category B.

Lioresal: see BACLOFEN

Lipo-Nicin: see NICOTINIC ACID

LISINOPRIL (Prinivil, Zestril; see also Prinzide, Zestoretic)

Dose: Initial, 10 mg PO qd (5 mg if patient is taking diuretics); usual, 10–40 mg PO qd.

Preparations: 5, 10, 20, and 40 mg tablets.

Actions: ACE inhibitor that causes vasodilatation; used to treat hypertension and CHF.

Clearance: No liver metabolism; 100% renal excreted.
Moderately reduce dosage in impaired renal function.

Side Effects: Hypotension, angioedema, oliguria or azotemia, nonproductive cough, hyperkalemia, BUN, and creatinine.

Cautions: Contraindicated during second and third trimesters of pregnancy.

Use with caution in patients taking K+-sparing drugs.

Pearls: Cost $$$–$$$$ (≈$2/d retail).

BP reduction is smaller than average in black patients.

Is potentiated by diuretics.

Has no withdrawal effect.

Can decrease WBCs (drop in WBCs has been a rare side effect of other ACE inhibitors).

Occasionally check CBC, especially in patients with collagen vascular disease.

Pregnancy category D.

LITHIUM CARBONATE

Dose: 30 mg/kg PO loading dose given in 3 divided doses; maintenance, 900 mg–1.5 g PO daily, divided into tid–qid doses with regular pills or bid doses with SR pills.

Preparations: 300 mg capsules; 300 mg tablets; 300 and 450 mg sustained-release tablets; syrup containing 300 mg/5 mL (1 tsp).

Actions: Psychotropic agent that alters intraneural metabolism of catecholamines and can affect Na+ transport in neural cells; used to treat manic episodes in patients with bipolar disorder.

Clearance: Renal excreted.

Slightly to moderately reduce dosage in impaired renal function.

No change in dosage needed for liver disease.

Supplemental dose suggested after HD or PD.

Side Effects: Fine hand tremor and many other CNS effects, polyuria, nephrogenic diabetes insipidus, nephrotic syndrome, leukocytosis, numerous cardiovascular effects.

Drug Interactions: NaHCO$_3$, acetazolamide, aminophylline, and osmotic diuretics all increase its excretion. Can potentiate response to tricyclics.

Cautions: Contraindicated in significant cardiovascular or renal disease, in Na+-depleted patients, in patients taking diuretics, and in pregnant or potentially pregnant patients.

Pearls: Cost $ (≈$8 retail/100 tablets).

Risk of toxicity is increased when serum level reaches 1.5–2.0 meq/L; some patients are unusually sensitive to lithium and can exhibit toxic signs at serum levels of 1.0–1.5 meq/L.

Symptoms of toxicity include diarrhea, vomiting, drowsiness, muscle weakness and incoordination, giddiness, ataxia, blurred vision, tinnitus, and large output of dilute urine.

Can significantly harm the fetus when administered during pregnancy.

Lodine: *see* ETODOLAC

Lomotil (DIPHENOXYLATE + ATROPINE)

Dose: 2 tablets or 2 tsp PO tid–qid until diarrhea is controlled, then 1 tablet or 1 tsp PO bid–tid.

Preparations: Tablets containing 2.5 mg diphenoxylate and 25 µg atropine; 2 oz bottles of liquid containing 2.5 mg diphenoxylate and 25 µg atropine per 5 mL (1 tsp).

Actions: Antidiarrheal agent with narcotic-like action that slows GI motility; used to treat diarrhea.

Side Effects: Numbness of extremities, depression, euphoria, drowsiness, angioedema, anaphylaxis, paralytic ileus, pancreatitis.

Cautions: Contraindicated in advanced liver disease and in patients taking MAOI.

Pearls: Cost: generic $, Lomotil $$$ (100 tablets retail: generic ≈$10, Lomotil ≈$40).

Pregnancy category C.

LOPERAMIDE (Imodium)

Dose: Initial, 2 capsules (4 mg), 2 caplets (4 mg), or 4 tsp (4 mg); then 1 capsule (2 mg), 1 caplet (2 mg), or 2 tsp (2 mg) after each unformed stool. Max, 16 mg PO daily.

Preparations: 6 and 12 tablet blister-packs containing 2 mg scored Imodium A-D caplets; 2 mg capsules; 2, 3, and 4 oz bottles of cherry-flavored liquid containing 1 mg/5 mL (1 tsp).

Actions: Antidiarrheal agent that slows GI peristalsis.

Clearance: Significant first-pass metabolism; excreted primarily in feces.

Side Effects: Rash, abdominal distress.

Cautions: Use with caution in liver dysfunction.

Pearls: Cost $$ (12 tablet blister-pack ≈$9 retail; ≈$65 retail/ 100 tablets).

Discontinue if abdominal distention occurs in patients with ulcerative colitis or pseudomembranous colitis (agents that inhibit intestinal motility have been reported to induce toxic megacolon).

Pregnancy category B.

Lopid: *see* GEMFIBROZIL

Lopressor: *see* METOPROLOL

Lorelco: *see* PROBUCOL

Losec: *see* OMEPRAZOLE

Lotensin: *see* BENAZEPRIL

Lotrimin: *see* CLOTRIMAZOLE

Lotrisone topical cream (CLOTRIMAZOLE + BETAMETHASONE)

Dose: Apply to skin bid.

Preparations: 15 and 45 g tubes.

Actions: Combination topical antifungal and steroid.

Pearls: Cost $$$ (15 g tube ≈$20 retail; 45 g tube ≈$36 retail).
Pregnancy category C.

LOVASTATIN (Mevacor)

Dose: Initial, 20 mg PO qd with evening meal; usual, 20–80 mg PO qd.

Allow at least 4 weeks before adjusting dosage.

Maximium dose in patients taking immunosuppressants, 20 mg daily.

Preparations: 10, 20, and 40 mg tablets.

Actions: HMG-CoA inhibitor that lowers cholesterol production, increasing HDL and reducing LDL, VLDL, and triglyceride levels; used to treat hypercholesterolemia.

Clearance: Hydrolyzed to active form.

No change in dosage needed in impaired renal function.

Side Effects: Elevated LFTs, increased CPK (MM) and myopathy (especially when given with immunosuppressants, gemfibrozil, or niacin), GI discomfort.

Drug Interactions: Can prolong PT in patients taking warfarin.

Cautions: Contraindicated in liver dysfunction and in pregnant or potentially pregnant patients.

Pearls: Cost $$$–$$$$ (≈$160 retail/100 tablets).

Obtain LFTs before starting therapy.

Recommended frequency for checking liver function during treatment has been liberalized to q6wk for first 3 months, then q8wk for remainder of first year and approximately every 6 months thereafter.

Discontinue if persistent LFTs >3 times normal, substantial rise in CPK, or myositis occurs.

Follow-up studies do *not* suggest increased incidence of lens opacification, so slit-lamp examinations appear unnecessary.

Pregnancy category X.

Lozol: see INDAPAMIDE

Maalox (MAGNESIUM HYDROXIDE + ALUMINUM HYDROXIDE)

Dose: 2–4 tablets or 2–4 tsp PO qid, given 60 min after meals and qhs.

Macrodantin: *see* NITROFURANTOIN

MAGNESIUM HYDROXIDE (MILK OF MAGNESIA, M.O.M.; *see also* Maalox, Mylanta, Rolaids)

Dose: 30 mL PO q6h prn.

Actions: Osmotic laxative; used to treat constipation or dyspepsia.

Pearls: Cost $.
Magnesium levels can markedly rise in patients with ESRD.
When taken as antacid, consider alternating with an aluminum-based antacid such as Amphogel or ALternaGEL (repeated use can cause diarrhea).

MAGNESIUM OXIDE (Mag-Ox 400)

Dose: 1–2 tablets PO qd.

Preparations: Bottles of 100 or 1000 tablets; each tablet contains 400 mg magnesium oxide.

Actions: Oral magnesium supplement.

Side Effects: Diarrhea.

Pearls: Cost $.
Signs and symptoms of hypomagnesemia include weakness, convulsions, and arrhythmias.

MAGNESIUM SULFATE

Dose: 1–2 g (8–16 meq magnesium) IV.

Preparations: 2 and 4 mg vials of 50% solution containing 8 or 16 meq magnesium, respectively.

Actions: IV magnesium supplement.

Mag-Ox: *see* MAGNESIUM OXIDE

Mandol: see CEFAMANDOLE

MANNITOL

Dose: 25–75 g or 1 g/kg of 20% solution IV; may repeat approximately q6h prn.

Actions: Osmotic agent that increases effective intravascular volume and diuresis.

Side Effects: Necrosis if extravasated.

Cautions: Use with caution in CHF.

Pearls: Watch for signs of CHF and pulmonary edema during use.

Maxzide, Maxzide-25 (TRIAMTERENE + HYDROCHLOROTHIAZIDE)

Dose: 1 tablet PO qd.

Preparations: Tablets containing 75 mg triamterine and 50 mg hydrochlorothiazide (Maxzide), or 37.5 mg triamterine and 25 mg hydrochlorothiazide (Maxzide-25).

Actions: Combination K^+-sparing diuretic; used to treat hypertension.

Clearance: Avoid in ESRD.
Reduce dosage in liver disease.

Side Effects: Hyperkalemia, dilutional hyponatremia, GI discomfort.

Drug Interactions: Increases risk of lithium toxicity. Heightens risk of renal failure when used with NSAID and of hyperkalemia when used with ACE inhibitors or K^+ supplements. Potentiates antihypertensive effects of other drugs.

Pearls: Cost $$ (100 tablets retail: 75/50 mg generic ≈$30, Maxzide ≈$65, Maxzide-25 ≈$37); no generic equivalent of Maxzide-25.
Pregnancy category C.

MECLIZINE (Antivert)

Dose: Disease dependent.
Vertigo: 25 mg PO tid–qid.
Motion sickness: 25–50 mg PO taken 1 h prior to embarkation; may be repeated q24h during trip.

Preparations: 12.5, 25, and 50 mg tablets; 25 mg chewable tablets.

Actions: Antihistamine; used to treat vertigo and motion sickness.

Side Effects: Drowsiness, dry mouth, blurred vision.

Cautions: Use with caution (because of anticholinergic actions) in asthma, glaucoma, or prostate hypertrophy.

Pearls: Cost: generic $, Antivert $$$ (100 tablets retail: 25 mg generic ≈$10, 25 mg Antivert ≈$50).
Pregnancy category B.

Medipren: see IBUPROFEN

Medrol: see METHYLPREDNISOLONE

MEDROXYPROGESTERONE (Provera)

Dose: Often given 5–10 mg PO qd with food, sometimes for 5–10 days. Dosing regimens vary significantly by disease.

Preparations: 2.5, 5, and 10 mg tablets; also available for IM injection.

Actions: Progesterone derivative that transforms estrogenic proliferative endometrium into secretory endometrium; used to treat secondary amenorrhea, abnormal uterine bleeding, and other conditions including respiratory acidosis and sleep apnea.

Clearance: Significant hepatic metabolism with 20–40% excreted in urine as metabolites, 5–15% excreted in stool.

Side Effects: Thrombotic disorders, menstrual irregularities, weight gain, rare breast tenderness or galactorrhea, rare skin reactions. Possibly associated with visual impairment.

Cautions: Contraindicated in patients with history of thrombophlebitis, thromboembolic disorders, liver disease, documented or suspected malignancy of breast or genital organs, vaginal bleeding of unknown cause, missed abortions, or cerebrovascular disease.
Contraindicated in pregnant and potentially pregnant patients.

Pearls: Cost $ ($\approx$$5 retail/100 tablets).
Can cause fetal damage during pregnancy.

Mefoxin: see CEFOXITIN

Mellaril, Mellaril-S: see THIORIDAZINE

MELPHALAN (Alkeran)

Dose: Regimens are somewhat variable; often, 6 mg PO qd for induction and 2 mg PO qd for maintenance.
For multiple myeloma, 0.25 mg/kg daily in 4-day cycles in combination with prednisone.
Should not be given with food.

Preparations: 2 mg scored tablets.

Actions: Alkylating agent; used treat neoplastic diseases.

Clearance: Metabolized via liver.
One source recommends no change in dosage for impaired renal function; another suggests 50% reduction in dose for BUN >30 or creatinine >1.5.

Side Effects: Myelosuppression, rare pulmonary fibrosis, rare GI distress and side effects, allergic hypersensitivity, increased incidence of secondary acute leukemia.

Pearls: Cost $$ ($\approx$$1/tablet wholesale).
Myelosuppression is dose-limiting toxicity.
WBC and platelet nadirs usually occur 14–21 days after treatment.
Pregnancy category D.

MEPERIDINE (Demerol)

Dose: 50–150 mg IM, SQ, or PO q3–4h.

Preparations: 50 and 100 mg tablets; 50 mg/5 mL (1 tsp) syrup; 10, 25, 50, 75, and 100 mg/mL injection.

Actions: Synthetic narcotic analgesic; used to treat pain.

Clearance: Metabolized predominantly via liver.
Normeperidine, an active and neurotoxic metabolite, can accumulate in ESRD and cause seizures.
Slightly reduce dosage in impaired renal function.
Decrease dosage in liver disease.

Side Effects: Respiratory depression, nausea and vomiting, hypotension, sweating, constipation (minor but common).

Cautions: Contraindicated in patients who have taken MAOI within 14 days.
Use with caution in respiratory or liver disease.
Can aggravate preexisting convulsive disorders.

Pearls: Cost $$$ (100 tablets retail: 50 mg generic ≈$33, 50 mg Demerol ≈$66, 100 mg generic ≈$50, 100 mg Demerol ≈$120; 5 mg IM $0.50).
Often given IM with Vistaril to decrease nausea (usually 50 mg Demerol with 25 mg Vistaril, or 75 or 100 mg Demerol with 50 mg Vistaril).
Can increase ventricular response in atrial flutter and other SVTs (because of vagolytic action).
Can raise serum levels of amylase and lipase.
50–80 mg meperidine has analgesic effect approximately equal to that of 10 mg morphine.
Pregnancy category not established.

MERCAPTOPURINE (6-MP, Purinethol)

Dose: 1.5–5.0 mg/kg PO qd.

Preparations: 50 mg scored tablets.

Actions: Purine-analog antimetabolite that interferes with nucleic acid synthesis; used to treat malignancies.

Clearance: Metabolized via liver to active metabolites.

No change in dosage needed for mild renal failure; may need to reduce dosage in patients with severely decreased CrCl.

Avoid in liver disease.

Side Effects: Myelosuppression, hepatotoxicity (both cholestasis and parenchymal injury). Nausea and vomiting occur rarely.

Drug Interactions: Allopurinol markedly decreases its catabolism. Trimethoprim + sulfamethoxazole (Bactrim, Septra) increases its bone marrow suppression.

Cautions: Reduce to 1/3 to 1/4 the normal dose when given with allopurinol.

Pearls: Cost $$ ($\approx$$6/d wholesale).

Pregnancy category D.

MESNA (Mesnex)

Dose: Used in conjunction with ifosfamide therapy. Administered as 3 injections, each at 20% of ifosfamide dose (in mg), as follows:

Give initial mesna dose concurrently with ifosfamide injection; repeat dose 4 and 8 h later (mesna total, 60% of ifosfamide dose). Repeat this dosing schedule each time ifosfamide is given.

Example: For 1.2 g/m^2 ifosfamide dose, give 240 mg/m^2 mesna simultaneously, another 240 mg/m^2 4 h later, and another 240 mg/m^2 8 h after initial injection.

Preparations: 2, 4, and 10 mL ampules containing 100 mg/mL.

Actions: Thiol agent that acts to detoxify urotoxic metabolites of ifosfamide in the kidneys; used as prophylaxis or antidote for ifosfamide-induced hemorrhagic cystitis.

Clearance: Oxidized in blood to its active metabolite mesna disulfide, which is renal excreted.

Side Effects: Nausea and vomiting, diarrhea.

Cautions: Contraindicated in patients with known allergies to thiol compounds.

Pearls: Cost $$ (400 mg ≈$28 wholesale).

May also be used with cyclophosphamide to reduce hemorrhagic cystitis.

Pregnancy category B.

Mesnex: see MESNA

MESTRANOL: see Norinyl, Ortho-Novum oral contraceptive pills

Metamucil (PSYLLIUM)

Dose: 1 rounded tsp in 8 oz liquid qd–tid.

Preparations: 7, 14, and 21 oz containers; cartons of 100 single-dose packets; available in sugar-free and "grit-free" preparations.

Actions: Bulk-forming fiber; used to restore and maintain bowel regularity.

Pearls: Cost $$ (container ≈$15 retail).

Can cause allergic reaction in patients sensitive to inhaled or ingested psyllium powder (consider using Citrucel).

Available in sugar-containing and sugar-free flavors including orange, lemon-lime, and strawberry.

Safe to use during pregnancy.

Metaprel: see METAPROTERENOL

METAPROTERENOL (Alupent, Metaprel)

Dose: Delivery dependent.

PO: 20 mg tid–qid.

Nebulizer: 0.3 mL of 5% solution in 2.5 mL NS.

Metered-dose inhaler: 2 or 3 inhalations q3–4h; max, 12 inhalations daily.

Preparations: 10 and 20 mg tablets; each Alupent inhalation aerosol contains 150 mg metaproterenol and delivers 200 inhalations; 10 mg/5 mL (1 tsp) cherry-flavored syrup; inhalation solution for nebulizers.

Actions: β-stimulating bronchodilator; used to treat reactive airway disease.

Side Effects: Tachycardia, palpitations, hypertension, nervousness, tremor, nausea and vomiting, bad taste.

Cautions: Use with caution in patients with CAD or tachyarrhythmias.

Pearls: Cost $$$ (Alupent or Metapril inhaler ≈$14–$20 retail; metaproterenol tablets ≈$0.10 each wholesale).
Pregnancy category C.

METHADONE

Dose: Disease dependent.
Pain: 2.5–10 mg PO, IM, or SQ q3–4h.
Drug detoxification: Initial, 15–20 mg PO, IM, or SQ; usual, 40 mg qd or 20 mg PO, IM, or SQ bid.

Preparations: 5 and 10 mg tablets; 5 and 10 mg/5 mL (1 tsp) oral solution; 10 mg/mL injection.

Actions: Synthetic narcotic analgesic; used to treat pain and for narcotic detoxification.

Clearance: Metabolized via liver.
Slightly decrease dosage in ESRD; no change needed for milder renal impairment.
Reduce dosage in liver disease.
Supplemental dose not required after HD or PD.

Side Effects: Respiratory depression, CNS changes, hypotension, urine retention, biliary tree spasm, antidiuretic effects.

Drug Interactions: Rifampin can decrease its serum level.

Cautions: Use with caution in patients taking other CNS depressants.

Pearls: Cost $ (10 mg ≈$16 retail/100 tablets).
Can produce drug dependence.
Methadone withdrawal, though qualitatively similar to morphine withdrawal, is of slower onset, has more prolonged course, and has less severe symptoms.
Is a schedule II controlled substance.
Is *not* an anxiolytic.
In overdose therapy, naloxone (Narcan) is effective for only 1–3 h while methadone is effective 36–48 h, so patients must be monitored for relapsing CNS depression when Narcan wears off.
Pregnancy category not established.

METHAZOLAMIDE (Neptazane)

Dose: 50–100 mg PO bid–tid with food.

Preparations: 25 and 50 mg tablets.

Actions: Carbonic anhydrase inhibitor that decreases production of aqueous humor; used to treat open-angle glaucoma.

Side Effects (systemic): Malaise, fatigue, depression, anorexia and weight loss, loss of libido, metabolic alkalosis.

Cautions: Use with caution in respiratory disease, renal disease, liver disease, adrenal insufficiency, hyperchloremic acidosis, hyponatremia or hypokalemia, and in patients with history of sulfa allergy.

Pearls: Cost $$$ (50 mg ≈$80 retail/100 tablets).
A urinary alkalinizing agent.
Pregnancy category C.

METHIMAZOLE (Tapazole)

Dose: Recommendations for initial dose vary: *PDR* recommends 5–20 mg PO q8h; other sources suggest single daily dose of 10–30 mg PO initially for mild disease.
Maintenance: 5–15 mg PO qd.
Consider consulting an endocrinologist for dosing recommendations.

Preparations: 5 and 10 mg tablets.

Actions: Medication that blocks synthesis of thyroid hormone by inhibiting iodide organification; used to treat hyperthyroidism.

Clearance: Rapidly metabolized.
No change in dosage needed for impaired renal function.

Side Effects: Agranulocytosis (dose related); decreased PMNs, platelets, and hematocrit; elevated LFTs, hepatitis, cholestatic jaundice, nephrotic syndrome, drug fever, SLE-like syndrome, insulin autoimmune syndrome (resulting in substantially reduced serum glucose and hypoglycemia), hypoprothrombinemia, loss of taste.

Drug Interactions: Potentiates anti-vitamin K activity of warfarin and can prolong PT in patients taking warfarin.

Pearls: Cost $$ (≈$0.30/d retail).
Monitor CBC.
Warn patients to report signs of infection.
Pregnancy category D.

METHOTREXATE

Dose: Tumor dependent. May be given PO, IV, or intrathecally.

Actions: Antimetabolite that inhibits dihydrofolate reductase, interfering with cell reproduction; used to treat malignancies, recalcitrant psoriasis, and rheumatoid arthritis.

Clearance: Route dependent: PO, hepatic and intracellularly metabolized to active metabolites; IV, 80%–90% excreted unchanged in urine with limited biliary excretion.
Moderately reduce dosage in impaired renal function; avoid in ESRD.
Use with caution in liver disease (because of hepatotoxicity).
Supplemental dose suggested after HD but not PD.

Side Effects: Ulcerative stomatitis, leukopenia, nausea and GI distress, malaise, fatigue, fever and chills, dizziness, decreased resistance to infections, hepatotoxicity, renal damage (when used in high doses for osteosarcoma).

Drug Interactions: ASA, NSAID, and probenecid decrease its tubular secretion and can increase its toxicity. ASA, phenytoin, and sulfonamides can displace protein-bound methotrexate and thus increase its toxicity. Trimethoprim + sulfamethoxazole (Bactrim, Septra) rarely can increase its bone marrow suppression (probably secondary to antifolate effects).

Cautions: Contraindicated for treatment of psoriasis in pregnant or potentially pregnant patients.

Pearls: Cost $$ (250 mg ≈$10 wholesale).
Coadministration of leucovorin decreases potential for toxicity with high-dose therapy.
Folate deficiency can increase its toxicity.
Accumulates in and exits slowly from third space fluid collections.
Periodically check CBC, LFTs, BUN, and creatinine.
For severe reactions or toxicity, consider giving leucovorin to counteract the metabolic effects of methotrexate and reduce the resulting toxicity (commonly referred to as "leucovorin rescue").
Pregnancy category X.

METHYLDOPA (Aldomet)

Dose: Initial, 250 mg PO bid–tid for first 48 h; usual, 500 mg–2 g daily PO given bid–qid; max, 3 g PO daily.

Preparations: 125, 250, and 500 mg tablets; 250 mg/5 mL (1 tsp) oral suspension.

Actions: Centrally acting agent; used to treat hypertension.

Clearance: Metabolized via liver; renal excreted.
Moderately increase dosing interval in impaired renal function.
Avoid in liver disease.
Supplemental dose suggested after HD or PD.

Side Effects: Sedation, headache, asthenia, depression, impotence, weakness, nasal congestion, (+) Coombs' reaction within 6–12 months (10%–20%). Occasional complex of fever, elevated LFTs, and eosinophilia. Occasional false (+) test for lupus, (+) rheumatoid factor, or (+) ANA titer.

Cautions: Contraindicated in active hepatic disease.

Pearls: Cost: generic $$, Aldomet $$$ (generic ≈$0.60/d retail, Aldomet ≈$1.50/d retail).

Frequently causes (+) Coombs' test but rarely causes hemolytic anemia.

May falsely elevate urinary catecholamine levels.

Paradoxical increase in BP can occur with IV use.

Pregnancy category B.

METHYLPREDNISOLONE (Depo-Medrol, Medrol, Solu-Medrol)

Dose: Preparation dependent.

Medrol: 4–48 mg PO qd.

Solu-Medrol: 60–125 mg IV q6h.

Depo-Medrol: Variable intra-articular dose (large joint 20–80 mg; medium joint 16–40 mg; small joint 4–10 mg); may also be given 80–120 mg IM for systemic therapy.

Preparations: 2, 4, 8, 16, 24, and 32 mg tablets; various preparations for injection. Medrol dose pack contains 4 mg Medrol tablets beginning with 6 tablets (24 mg) the first day and tapering daily dose by 1 tablet (4 mg) each day over 6 days.

Actions: Corticosteroid with anti-inflammatory properties; used primarily to treat inflammatory and allergic conditions.

Clearance: Metabolized via liver.

No change in dosage needed for impaired renal function.

Dosage adjustment probably not needed in liver disease.

Supplemental dose suggested after HD.

Side Effects: Mild NaCl and water retention (which can lead to increased hypertension, edema, and CHF), increased glucose intolerance and catabolism, decreased wound healing. Can aggravate peptic ulcer disease.

Pearls: Cost: generic $, Medrol $$ (dose pack: generic ≈$6 retail, Medrol ≈$13 retail).

Patients may need "stress steroids" during chronic therapy.

Can mask signs of infection.

In one study, IV administration improved prognosis in patients with acute spinal cord trauma and neurologic changes who were treated within 4 h of injury. The protocol was: (1) 30 mg bolus administered over 15 min, then continuous infusion of 5.4 mg/kg/h for 23 h (*NEJM*, May 1990).

Pregnancy category not established; observe newborns for hypoadrenalism.

Relative steroid activity:

	Relative anti-inflammatory and glucocorticoid activity	*Relative mineralocorticoid activity*
methylprednisolone	5.0	0.5
hydrocortisone	1.0	1.0
prednisone	4.0	0.8
dexamethasone	25–30	0.0

METOCLOPRAMIDE (Reglan)

Dose: Disease dependent.

GE reflux: 10–15 mg PO qid (5 mg in sensitive elderly patients) given 30 min before meals and qhs for 4–12 weeks.

Diabetic gastroparesis: 10 mg PO, IM, or IV given 30 min before each meal and qhs for 2–8 weeks.

Chemotherapy-induced nausea and vomiting: 1–2 mg/kg given over 15 min starting 30 min before chemotherapy; repeat dose 2, 5, 8, and 11 h after first dose.

Preparations: 5 and 10 mg tablets; 5 mg/5 mL (1 tsp) syrup; 5 mg vials.

Actions: Medication with central antidopaminergic and peripheral cholinergic properties that increases lower esophageal sphincter tone, enhances upper GI motility, and antagonizes dopamine-mediated nausea and vomiting; used to treat esophageal reflux and diabetic gastroparesis and to prevent chemotherapy-induced nausea and vomiting.

Clearance: Metabolized via liver; renal excreted.

Slightly reduce dosage in impaired renal function; extrapyramidal reactions are common in ESRD.

No change in dosage needed for liver disease.
Supplemental dose not required after HD or PD.

Side Effects: Tardive dyskinesia, acute dystonic reactions, Parkinson-like symptoms, drowsiness, depression, confusion.

Drug Interactions: Concomitant use with MAOI causes hypertensive crisis. Phenothiazines increase risk of extrapyramidal events. Anticholinergics and narcotics decrease its GI motility effects and narcotics increase its CNS depression. Decreases absorption of drugs absorbed in the stomach (e.g., digoxin) and increases absorption of drugs absorbed in the small intestine.

Cautions: Contraindicated in GI bleeding, gastric outlet or intestinal obstruction, epilepsy, pheochromocytoma, and in patients taking MAOI or drugs likely to cause extrapyramidal reactions. Use with caution in hypertensive patients (can cause release of catecholaminese when given IV).

Pearls: Cost: generic $$, Reglan $$$$ (PO: generic ≈$0.70/d retail, Reglan ≈$2/d retail; 20 mg IV ≈$2 wholesale).
Extrapyramidal reactions can be treated with a single dose of diphenhydramine (Benadryl) 50 mg IM.
Pregnancy category B.

METOLAZONE (Zaroxolyn)

Dose: Disease dependent.
Edema: 5–20 mg PO qd.
Hypertension: 2.5–5 mg PO qd.

Preparations: 2.5, 5, and 10 mg tablets.

Actions: Quinazoline diuretic that affects electrolyte absorption in the renal tubules, similar to action of thiazides; used to treat CHF and edema, often in conjunction with furosemide.

Clearance: Predominantly excreted unchanged in urine.
No change in dosage needed for impaired renal function; avoid in ESRD.
No change in dosage required for liver disease.
Supplemental dose not required after HD.

Side Effects: Hypokalemia K^+, increased glucose and uric acid.

Cautions: Contraindicated in anuria, hepatic coma, and gout.

Pearls: Cost $$ (≈$60 retail/100 tablets); no generic form available.

Unlike thiazides, can produce diuresis in patients with GFR <20 mL/min.

Often works synergistically with furosemide.

Can reactivate latent SLE.

Pregnancy category B.

METOPROLOL (Lopressor, Toprol XL)

Dose: Route dependent.

PO: 50–100 mg bid of Lopressor; 50–200 mg PO qd of long-acting Toprol XL.

IV (in acute MI): 5 mg Lopressor q5min for total of 15 mg (as tolerated).

Preparations: Lopressor: 50 and 100 mg tablets; 1 mg/mL injection; Toprol XL: 50, 100, and 200 long-acting tablets.

Actions: β_1-Selective β-blocker; used to treat angina and hypertension.

Clearance: Metabolized via liver.

No change in dosage needed for impaired renal function.

Supplemental dose suggested after HD.

Side Effects: Decreased ejection fraction, hypotension, CHF, AV block, bradycardia, diarrhea, rash, pruritus, bronchospasm, depression, disorientation, impotence.

Cautions: Relatively contraindicated in sinus bradycardia, >first-degree AV block, PR interval >0.24 sec, severely decreased ejection fraction, and bronchospastic disease.

Pearls: Cost $$ (100 tablets retail: 50 mg PO Lopressor ≈$40, 100 mg PO Lopressor ≈$60, 100 mg PO Toprol XL ≈$85; 5 mg IV Lopressor ≈$5 wholesale).

Taper dose when discontinuing to avoid rebound reactions.

Pregnancy category C.

METRONIDAZOLE (Flagyl)

Dose: Disease dependent.
Trichomoniasis: 2 g PO single dose, or 250 mg PO tid for 7 days.
Intestinal amebiasis: 750 mg PO tid for 5 days.
Giardiasis: 250 mg PO tid for 5 days.
C. difficile infection: 250 mg PO or IV tid for 7 days.
Serious infection: 500 mg IV q6–8h.

Preparations: 250 and 500 mg tablets; 500 mg vials for injection.

Actions: Antibiotic used to treat anaerobic bacterial infections and amebiasis, giardiasis, trichomoniasis, and *Gardnerella vaginalis* infections.

Clearance: Metabolized via liver; renal excreted.
Slightly decrease dosage in ESRD (metabolites can rarely cause an SLE-like syndrome); no change needed for milder renal impairment.
Reduce dosage in liver dysfunction.
Supplemental dose suggested after HD but not after PD.

Side Effects: GI discomfort, mild decrease in WBCs, Antabuse-like reaction if mixed with alcohol, peripheral neuropathy and seizures (immediately discontinue for either), pseudomembranous colitis.

Drug Interactions: Prolongs PT in patients taking warfarin. Raises serum level of lithium. Induces hepatic enzymes. Cimetidine decreases its serum level.

Pearls: Cost: generic $$, Flagyl $$$ (1 week of therapy: generic ≈$10 retail, Flagyl ≈$30 retail).
Can interfere with laboratory assays of alanine and aspartate transaminase (ALT, AST), lactate dehydrogenase, and triglycerides.
Excellent abscess penetration.
Penicillin or clindamycin is preferred for aspiration pneumonia (metronidazole does not cover microaerophilic streptococcus, one of the anaerobic organisms associated with aspiration pneumonia).

Warn patients to avoid alcohol ingestion during use.

Long-term use (i.e., in Crohn's disease) is associated with peripheral neuropathy.

Pregnancy category B.

Mevacor see LOVASTATIN

MEXILETINE (Mexitil)

Dose: 200–400 mg PO tid with meals.

Preparations: 150, 200, and 250 mg capsules.

Actions: Type Ib antiarrhythmic; used to treat ventricular arrhythmias.

Clearance: Metabolized via liver; 33% renal excreted.

Slightly reduce dosage in ESRD; no change needed for milder renal impairment.

Increase dosing interval to q24h or longer in liver disease.

Supplemental dose suggested after HD but not PD.

Side Effects: Palpitations, chest pain, nausea and vomiting, elevated LFTs, heartburn, light-headedness, dizziness, tremor, ataxia, coordination difficulties, visual changes, mental status changes.

Drug Interactions: Can raise serum level of theophylline. Cimetidine can raise or lower its serum level. Hepatic enzyme inducing drugs (phenytoin, phenobarbital, rifampin, etc.) decrease its serum level.

Pearls: Cost $$$$ (>$2.50/d retail).

Usual therapeutic level is 0.5–2.0 µg/mL.

Pregnancy category C.

Mexitil: see MEXILETINE

Mezlin: see MEZLOCILLIN

MEZLOCILLIN (Mezlin)

Dose: 3 g IV q4h or 4 g IV q6h.

Actions: Bactericidal antipseudomonal penicillin that inhibits cell wall synthesis. Some gram (+) coverage including enterococci and strep (but *not* staph); excellent gram (−) coverage including *P. aeruginosa;* good anaerobic coverage including *B. fragilis.*

Clearance: Primarily renal excreted; some hepatobiliary excretion.
  Slightly increase dosing interval in impaired renal function.
  No change in dosage needed for liver disease.
  Supplemental dose not required after HD or PD.

Side Effects: Rash, drug fever, anaphylactic reactions, interstitial nephritis, GI distress, elevated LFTs, seizures (with excessive dose), leukopenia, eosinophilia, thrombocytopenia, phlebitis.

Drug Interactions: Probenecid raises its serum level.

Pearls: Cost $$$ (4 g $15 wholesale).
  Contains high Na^+ load.
  Pregnancy category B.

MICONAZOLE (Monistat Vaginal Suppositories, Monistat Vaginal Cream)

Dose: Route dependent.
  Cream: Apply qhs for 7 days (for Monistat 7).
  Suppository: Insert intravaginally qhs for 3 days (Monistat 3) or 7 days (Monistat 7).

Preparations: 1.59 oz tubes of Monistat 7 Vaginal Cream; 200 mg Monistat 3 Vaginal Suppositories; 100 mg Monistat 7 Vaginal Suppositories.

Actions: Fungicidal antibiotic; used to treat *Candida* vaginitis.

Side Effects: Vulvovaginal burning, itching, or irritation, contact dermatitis.

Cautions: Should be avoided when possible during first trimester of pregnancy (orally absorbed miconazole has been shown to have fetotoxic effects in animals).

Pearls: Cost $$ (Monistat 3 ≈$24 retail; Monistat 7 ≈$17 retail; Monistat Cream ≈$17 retail).

Try to avoid in first trimester of pregnancy.

Micro-K: see POTASSIUM CHLORIDE

Micronase: see GLYBURIDE

Midamor: see AMILORIDE

MIDAZOLAM (Versed)

Dose: For preprocedure sedation and anesthesia, 0.15–0.35 mg/kg IV (approximately 1–2.5 mg for a 70 kg patient) injected over at least 20–30 sec. May give further small doses after at least 2 min.

Preparations: 1, 2, 5, and 10 mL vials containing 5 mg/mL Versed.

Actions: Short-acting benzodiazepine; used in induction of anesthesia and as sedative before procedures such as endoscopy or intubation.

Side Effects: Respiratory depression, apnea, pain at injection site, phlebitis.

Cautions: Should be used only by experienced personnel (because of potential for respiratory arrest).

Pearls: Cost $ (2 mg $3.60 wholesale).

Titrate *slowly* (some patients may respond to as little as 1 mg).

Always have oxygen and resuscitative equipment immediately available.

Impairs memory of periprocedure events.

Pregnancy category D.

MILK OF MAGNESIA: see MAGNESIUM HYDROXIDE

MINERAL OIL

Dose: Delivery dependent.
  PO: 15–45 mL qd–bid.
  Enema: 60–120 mg.

Preparations: 16 oz bottles.

Actions: Lubricant laxative; used to treat constipation.

Cautions: Should not be used with surfactant-type stool softeners.

Pearls: Cost $.
  Onset of action is 48–72 h with PO therapy, immediate when given as enema.
  Decreases absorption of fat-soluble vitamins.

Minipress: see PRAZOSIN

Minitran: see NITROGLYCERIN patch

MINOXIDIL topical solution (Rogaine)

Dose: Apply 1 mL of solution to scalp bid; max, 2 mL bid.

Preparations: 60 mL bottle containing 2% solution (20 mg/mL).

Actions: Topical agent that stimulates vertex hair growth and stabilizes hair loss; used to treat male-pattern baldness.

Side Effects: No increase in systemic effects compared with placebo.

Pearls: Cost $$$ (60 mL bottle $42 wholesale).
  Causes significant hair growth in only modest percentage of patients.
  Many patients need at least 4–8 months of treatment before achieving significant results.
  Remind patients who apply preparation with the fingers to wash hands after each use.
  Pregnancy category C.

MISOPROSTOL (Cytotec)

Dose: 200 μg PO qid with food; may give 100 μg PO qid if higher dose is not tolerated.

Preparations: 100 and 200 μg tablets.

Actions: Prostaglandin analog; used to prevent gastric ulcers in patients at high risk of complications from therapy with NSAID (including ASA); does *not* prevent duodenal ulcers or the GI pain and discomfort that can be associated with NSAID use.

Clearance: De-esterified to the active compound misoprostol acid, which is primarily renal excreted.

Dosage change not routinely needed for impaired renal function, but may be decreased if 200 μg dose is not tolerated.

Side Effects: Diarrhea, abdominal pain, nausea and vomiting, flatulence, headache, possible miscarriage, uterine bleeding.

Cautions: Contraindicated in patients with history of allergy to prostaglandins and in pregnant or potentially pregnant patients.

Pearls: Cost $$$$ (≈$2.50/d retail).

Pregnancy category X.

MITOMYCIN (MITOMYCIN-C, MTC, Mutamycin)

Dose: 20 mg/m^2 IV.

Preparations: 5, 20, and 40 mg vials that also contain mannitol.

Actions: Antibiotic that inhibits DNA synthesis; used to treat neoplastic diseases.

Clearance: Primarily metabolized in liver and other tissues; approximately 10%–30% excreted unchanged in urine.

Recommendations vary on need to adjust dosage in renal failure: one source notes it should not be used if serum creatinine >1.7 mg/dL; another source states no change is needed for CrCl >10 mL/min.

No change in dosage needed for liver disease.

Side Effects: Myelosuppression, nausea and vomiting, anorexia, diarrhea, alopecia, nephrotoxicity, stomatitis, fever, rare pulmonary toxicity, hemolytic-uremic syndrome, severe local irritation if extravasated.

Drug Interactions: Concurrent use with vinca alkaloids is associated with shortness of breath and severe bronchospasm.

Pearls: Cost $$$$ (40 mg $720 wholesale).
Myelosuppression is dose-limiting toxicity.
Average time for WBC and platelet nadirs is 4 weeks but can be as long as 8 weeks after therapy.
Pregnancy category not established.

MODURETIC (AMILORIDE + HYDROCHLOROTHIAZIDE)

Dose: 1 or 2 tablets PO qd (can be given bid).

Preparations: Each tablet contains 5 mg amiloride and 50 mg hydrochlorothiazide.

Actions: Combination K^+-sparing diuretic; used to treat hypertension.

Clearance: Avoid in ESRD.

Side Effects: Hyperkalemia, headache, dizziness, weakness, GI discomfort.

Drug Interactions: Concomitant use with indomethacin causes elevated K^+ level. Increases risk of lithium toxicity. Augments antihypertensive effects of other drugs.

Pearls: Cost $$ (100 tablets retail: generic ≈$25, Moduretic ≈$40).
Pregnancy category B.

M.O.M.: see MAGNESIUM HYDROXIDE

Monistat: see MICONAZOLE

Monopril: see FOSINOPRIL

MORICIZINE (Ethmozine)

Dose: Usual, 200–300 mg PO tid. Some patients may achieve arrhythmia control with bid dose.

Preparations: 200, 250, and 300 mg tablets.

Actions: Class I antiarrhythmic; used to treat life-threatening arrhythmias.

Clearance: Extensively metabolized; metabolites excreted in feces and urine.

Although no active metabolites are known to be renal excreted, it is recommended that patients with impaired renal function be started on a lower dose and carefully monitored.

Reduce dosage in liver dysfunction.

Side Effects: Dizziness, nausea, headache, proarrhythmic actions, conduction defects, numbness.

Cautions: Contraindicated in second- or third-degree AV block unless a pacemaker is in place.

May be contraindicated in bifascicular block unless a pacemaker is present.

Use with extreme caution in sick sinus syndrome (can cause sinus bradycardia, sinus pause or arrest, or conduction problems).

Pearls: Cost $$$$ ($\approx$$2–$3/d retail).

Increased mortality in certain patients when used to treat post-MI PVCs in the CAST study.

Discontinue if second- or third-degree heart block develops unless a pacemaker is in place.

Correct K^+ and Mg^{ff} abnormalities before beginning treatment.

Pregnancy category B.

MORPHINE (MS Contin)

Dose: Highly variable.

Initial, 2 mg IV, or 5–10 mg SQ, or 5–10 mg IM, or 5–20 mg PO; maintenance variable, with PO, SQ, and IM usually given q4h.

Controlled-release PO (MS Contin): Divide total daily dose into either halves or thirds and give q12h or q8h, respectively.

Acute MI: May give 2–4 mg IV at frequent intervals (avoid IM injections, which will elevate CPK levels).

IV drip may vary between 1–4 mg/h or significantly more, especially in cancer patients.

When converting from IV to PO, estimates of PO equivalent vary; *PDR* suggests that 3 times the IV dose may be sufficient. Titrate to pain.

Consider using lower initial and maintenance doses in elderly patients and in patients with respiratory or liver disease.

Preparations: 10, 15, and 30 mg tablets; 15, 30, 60, and 100 mg tablets of MS Contin (many pharmacies do not carry 15 mg tablets); 10, 20, and 100 mg/5 mL (1 tsp) solution; 5, 10, and 20 mg suppositories; 2, 4, 5, 8, and 15 mg/mL injection.

Actions: Narcotic analgesic that also promotes venous and arterial dilatation and reduces sensation of dyspnea; used to relieve pain and in acute treatment of CHF and pulmonary edema (if respiratory depression is not significant concern).

Clearance: Metabolized via liver; $t_{1/2}$ is prolonged in liver dysfunction.

Slightly decrease dosage in impaired renal function.

Reduce dosage in liver disease.

Supplemental dose not required after HD.

Side Effects: Substantial reduction in BP, respiratory depression, decreased pulmonary vascular resistance, nausea and vomiting, constipation, ileus, urine retention, sedation, hallucinations, withdrawal symptoms.

Pearls: Cost $, MS Contin $$$$ (100 tablets retail: 30 mg MS Contin ≈$120, 60 mg MS Contin ≈$230).

Can cause mast cell degranulation and histamine release.

Never crush tablets for administration via NG tube or for any other reason (may cause rapid absorption of high morphine doses).

Pregnancy category C.

Motrin, Motrin IB: *see* **IBUPROFEN**

6-MP: *see* **MERCAPTOPURINE**

MS Contin: *see* **MORPHINE**

MTC: see MITOMYCIN

Mucomyst: see ACETYLCYSTEINE

Mutamycin: see MITOMYCIN

Mycelex: see CLOTRIMAZOLE

Mycostatin: see NYSTATIN

Mydriacyl: see TROPICAMIDE

Mylanta (ALUMINUM HYDROXIDE, MAGNESIUM HYDROXIDE + SIMETHICONE)

Dose: 1 or 2 tablets or tsp, or 15–30 mg, between meals and qhs.

Myleran: see BUSULFAN

Mylicon: see SIMETHICONE

Mysoline: see PRIMIDONE

NABUMETONE (Relafen)

Dose: 500–2000 mg PO qd; usual, 1000 mg PO given in 1 dose at night.

Preparations: 500 and 750 mg tablets.

Actions: Nonsteroidal anti-inflammatory agent; used to treat arthritis.

Clearance: Undergoes biotransformation in liver to active metabolite 6-MNA, which is metabolized via liver to inactive products.
  Reduce dosage in severe renal disease.
  Dosage adjustment probably not needed in liver disease.
  Supplemental dose not required after HD.

Side Effects: Diarrhea, dyspepsia, abdominal pain, nausea, constipation, flatulence, (+) stool guaiac, rash, possible fluid retention and worsening of CHF, possible worsening of kidney function.

Cautions: Contraindicated in patients with salicylate sensitivity.

Although it may cause less upper GI bleeding or ulcers than other NSAID, still use with caution in patients with history of ulcer or upper GI bleeding.

Its use during third trimester of pregnancy may cause premature closure of the ductus arteriosus.

Pearls: Cost $$$.

One study suggests that although the incidence of subjective GI symptoms is similar, it may produce less endoscopically determined upper GI ulceration than other NSAID.

Pregnancy category C.

N-ACETYLCYSTEINE: see ACETYLCYSTEINE

NADOLOL (Corgard)

Dose: Initial, 40 mg PO qd; usual, 40–80 mg PO qd. Max, 160–240 mg qd for angina, 240–320 mg qd for hypertension.

Preparations: 40, 80, 120, and 160 mg tablets.

Actions: Nonselective β-blocker; used to treat hypertension and angina.

Clearance: Renal excreted.

Moderately reduce dosage in impaired renal function; significant accumulation can occur in ESRD.

No change in dosage needed for liver disease.

Supplemental dose suggested after HD.

Side Effects: Bradycardia, CHF, decreased BP, rare but potentially serious bronchospasm.

Drug Interactions: Has additive effect with catecholamine-depleting drugs. Can raise or depress serum glucose level in patients taking antidiabetic drugs.

Cautions: Contraindicated in bronchial asthma, sinus bradycardia, second- or third-degree heart block, or overt cardiac failure.

Pearls: Cost $$$ (40 mg ≈$75 retail/100 tablets).
Taper dose when discontinuing (to avoid rebound reactions).
Pregnancy category C.

NALOXONE (Narcan)

Dose: 0.4 mg (1 mL ampule or 1 mL prefilled syringe) IV, IM, or SQ; may repeat dose q2–3min up to 10 mg. May be given IM or SQ if no IV access is available.

Preparations: 1 mL ampules containing 0.4 mg/mL; 2 mL vials containing 1.0 mg/mL; 1 and 2 mL prefilled syringes containing 1.0 mg/mL.

Actions: Narcotic antagonist that reverses opioid effects, including respiratory depression, sedation, and hypotension; used to treat narcotic overdose.

Clearance: Metabolized via liver; renal excreted.

Side Effects: Abrupt reversal of narcotic depression can cause nausea and vomiting, sweating, elevated HR and BP, tremulousness, seizures and cardiac arrest, or increased PTT.

Pearls: Onset of action is 1–2 min when given IV, 3–5 min when given IM or SQ.
Reevaluate diagnosis of narcotic overdose if symptoms are not reversed after total of 10 mg.
Duration of action of some narcotics can exceed that of naloxone, so repeat dose and monitor as necessary.
In overdose therapy, naloxone is effective for only 1–3 h while many narcotic agents have significantly longer duration of action, so patients must be continuously monitored for relapsing signs and symptoms of overdose.
Pregnancy category B.

NAPHAZOLINE: see Naphcon-A

Naphcon-A ophthalmic solution (NAPHAZOLINE + PHENIRAMINE)

Dose: 1 drop (written "gtt") in the eye up to q3–4h.

Preparations: 5 and 15 mL solutions containing 0.025% naphazoline and 0.3% pheniramine.

Actions: Ophthalmic solution used to treat ocular irritation, congestion, and allergic or inflammatory conditions.

Cautions: Contraindicated in patients taking MAOI.

Pearls: Cost: generic $, Naphcon-A $$ (15 mL retail: generic ≈$11, Naphcon-A ≈$18).
  Pregnancy category not established.

Naprosyn: see NAPROXEN

NAPROXEN (Naprosyn)

Dose: 250–500 mg PO bid with food or antacids.

Preparations: 250, 375, and 500 mg tablets.

Actions: Nonsteroidal anti-inflammatory agent with analgesic and antipyretic action; used to treat inflammation and pain.

Clearance: Metabolized via liver.
  No change in dosage needed for impaired renal function.
  Supplemental dose not required after HD.

Side Effects: GI irritation and upper GI bleeding, proteinuria, interstitial nephritis, nephrotic syndrome, worsening of "prerenal" renal failure, reversible decrease in platelet aggregation, prolonged bleeding time.

Cautions: Contraindicated in patients with salicylate sensitivity or history of upper GI bleeding or ulcer.
  Can cause premature closure of the ductus arteriosus or complications during delivery when used during last trimester of pregnancy.

Pearls: Cost $$$ (500 mg ≈$100 retail/100 tablets).
Can cause Na^+ retention.
Should not be used during third trimester of pregnancy.

Narcan: see NALOXONE

Nasacort: see TRIAMCINOLONE nasal inhaler

Nasalcrom: see CROMOLYN SODIUM

Nebupent: see PENTAMIDINE

Nembutal: see PENTOBARBITAL

NEOMYCIN SULFATE (see also Cortisporin, Neosporin)

Dose: Disease or use dependent.
Hepatic encephalopathy: 1–2 g PO or via NG tube q4–6h.
Preop: 1 g PO.

Preparations: 500 mg tablets; 125 mg/5 mL (1 tsp) oral solution.

Actions: Poorly absorbed aminoglycoside that decreases production of NH_4 by GI bacteria; used to treat hepatic encephalopathy.

Side Effects: Nausea and vomiting. Some systemic absorption can increase risk of ototoxicity or nephrotoxicity in patients with renal dysfunction.

Drug Interactions: Can increase neuromuscular blockade if absorbed.

Pearls: Cost $ (≈$2/d wholesale).

Neosporin cream (POLYMYXIN B + NEOMYCIN)

Dose: Apply to skin qd–tid.

Preparations: 0.5 oz tubes.

Actions: Topical antibiotic mixture; used to prevent skin infections.

Side Effects: Skin sensitization, ototoxicity, nephrotoxicity.

Neo-Synephrine: see PHENYLEPHRINE

Neptazane: see METHAZOLAMIDE

Neupogen: see GRANULOCYTE COLONY-STIMULATING FACTOR

Neutra-Phos: see PHOSPHORUS

NIACIN: see NICOTINIC ACID

NICARDIPINE (Cardene)

Dose: 20–40 mg PO tid.

Preparations: 20 and 30 mg tablets.

Actions: Calcium-channel blocker; used to treat hypertension, angina, and systolic dysfunction.

Clearance: >99% metabolized via liver, but serum level is elevated in impaired renal function and is exponentially increased at higher doses.

Use with caution in mild liver disease; reduce dosage or increase dosing interval in severe liver disease.

Side Effects: Hypotension, reflex tachycardia, dizziness, headache, pedal edema, flushing. Can rarely increase angina.

Drug Interactions: Usually does not raise serum level of digoxin. Cimetidine increases its serum level.

Pearls: Cost $$$$ ($\approx$$2/d retail).
May have less ($-$) inotropic effect than nifedipine.
Pregnancy category C.

Nicobid: *see* NICOTINIC ACID

Nicoderm: *see* NICOTINE transdermal patch

Nicolar: *see* NICOTINIC ACID

NICOTINE transdermal patch (Habitrol, Nicoderm)

Dose: Preparation dependent.

Habitrol: For most patients, manufacturer recommends beginning with 21 mg/d patch with a new patch applied each day for 4–8 weeks; then decrease to a new 14 mg/d patch applied each day for 2–4 weeks; then decrease to a new 7 mg/d patch applied each day for 2–4 weeks; then discontinue.

Nicoderm: For most patients, manufacturer recommends using a new 21 mg/d patch applied each day for 6 weeks; then decrease to a new 14 mg/d patch applied each day for 2 weeks; then decrease to a new 7 mg/d patch applied each day for 2 weeks; then discontinue.

Patients who weigh <100 lb, smoke <10 cigarettes daily, or have history of cardiovascular disease should begin with the 14 mg/d patch for 4–8 weeks, then decrease to the 7 mg/d patch for 2–4 weeks.

Patches should be applied to a nonhairy, clean, and dry skin site on trunk or upper outer arm. After 24 h, patch should be removed and a new patch applied to a *different* site; the same skin site should not be used again for at least 7 days.

Preparations: Transdermal patches delivering 21, 14, or 7 mg/d of nicotine.

Actions: Transdermal system that delivers nicotine; used for prophylactic treatment of nicotine withdrawal in patients attempting to stop smoking.

Clearance: Metabolized via liver; renal excreted.

Side Effects: Local irritation, pruritus or erythema, diarrhea, dyspepsia, arthralgia or myalgia, somnolence, tachycardia. Nicotine toxicity is characterized by nausea and vomiting, diarrhea, abdominal pain, diaphoresis, flushing, dizziness, disturbed hearing and vision, confusion, weakness, palpitations, altered respiration, and hypotension.

Cautions: Contraindicated in patients with serious arrhythmias, severe or worsening angina, and in the immediate post-MI period.

Should not be used by patients <16 years old or by pregnant patients.

Use with caution in patients with peptic ulcer disease (nicotine delays healing), accelerated hypertension (nicotine increases risk of malignant hypertension), hyperthyroidism, diabetes, or pheochromocytoma (nicotine causes release of catecholamines by the adrenal medulla).

Pearls: Cost $$$ (≈$120/mo retail).

Patients who stop smoking may require reduction in dosage of imipramine, oxazepam, theophylline, insulin, prazosin, or labetalol.

Patients who continue to smoke while using the patch may experience increased side effects from elevated serum nicotine levels, possibly including myocardial infarction.

Warn patients to dispose of patches carefully so that children and pets do not apply or ingest discarded patches (residual nicotine remains on the patch after 24 h).

Pregnancy category D.

NICOTINIC ACID (Lipo-Nicin, Niacin, Nicobid, Nicolar, SloNiacin)

Dose: Initial, 100 mg PO tid with meals; gradually increase to 1–2 g PO tid. Usual dose of Slo-Niacin is one 750 mg tablet bid.

Preparations: 20, 25, 50, 100, and 500 mg tablets; 250, 500, and 750 mg tablets of Slo-Niacin.

Actions: Medication that inhibits synthesis of VLDL and decreases HDL catabolism, leading to reduced LDL and triglyceride and increased HDL levels.

Clearance: Metabolized via liver; renal excreted.

Moderately reduce dosage in impaired renal function; toxic reactions are frequent in ESRD.

Side Effects: Frequent flushing and pruritus (may decrease over time), GI discomfort, occasional jaundice, elevated LFTs, increased glucose and uric acid, hypotension.

Drug Interactions: Adrenergic blocking drugs can substantially increase peripheral vasodilatation, causing postural hypotension.

Cautions: Contraindicated in liver dysfunction, active peptic ulcer, arterial bleeding, and in patients with known idiosyncratic drug reactions.
Use with caution in gout or diabetes.

Pearls: Cost: generic $, brands $$$ (100 tablets retail: 500 mg generic ≈$10, 500 mg Nicobid ≈$75).
Aspirin or other NSAID taken 30 min before each dose can decrease flushing.
Pregnancy category not established.

NIFEDIPINE (Procardia, Procardia XL)

Dose: Preparation dependent.
Regular tablets: 10–40 mg PO tid.
Long-acting tablets: 30–90 mg PO qd of Procardia XL.
For elderly patients beginning therapy with regular tablets, give initial 5 mg test dose, at night if possible.

Preparations: 10, 20, and 30 mg tablets; 30, 60, and 90 mg long-acting tablets of Procardia XL.

Actions: Calcium-channel blocker; used to treat angina and hypertension.

Clearance: Metabolized via liver.
No change in dosage needed for impaired renal function.
Reduce dosage in liver disease.
Supplemental dose not required after HD.

Side Effects: Hypotension, dizziness or light-headedness, peripheral edema, flushing, reflex tachycardia anxiety, headache, rare (+) direct Coombs' reaction.

Drug Interactions: Can raise serum level of digoxin. Cimetidine increases its serum level.

Pearls: Cost $$$ (60 mg Procardia XL ≈$65 retail/100 tablets).
May give 10 mg PO or SL for urgent treatment of hypertension (physicians differ on whether sublingual administration produces quicker effect).
Pregnancy category C.

NIMODIPINE (Nimotop)

Dose: For subarachnoid hemorrhage: 60 mg PO q4h for 21 days.

Preparations: 30 mg tablets.

Actions: Calcium-channel blocker; used to prevent vasospasm in subarachnoid hemorrhage.

Clearance: Metabolized via liver.
Reduce dosage (to 30 mg q4h) in liver failure.

Side Effects: Hypotension, headache, flushing.

Drug Interactions: Can potentiate other antihypertensive agents.

Pearls: Cost $$$$ (≈$450 retail/100 tablets).
Start ASAP (within 96 h) after subarachnoid hemorrhage.
No IV form available; give via NG tube when necessary.
Pregnancy category C.

Nimotop: *see* **NIMODIPINE**

Nipride: *see* **NITROPRUSSIDE**

Nitro-Dur: *see* **NITROGLYCERIN patch**

NITROFURANTOIN (Macrodantin)

Dose: Disease dependent. Should be taken with food (to increase absorption).
Uncomplicated urinary tract infection: 50 mg PO qid.
Many other infections: 50–100 mg PO qid.

Preparations: 25, 50, and 100 mg capsules.

Actions: Bacteriostatic antibiotic that presumed to interfere with several bacterial enzyme systems; used to treat urinary tract infections. Good coverage of most organisms that cause these infections, including enterococci and staph.

Clearance: Metabolized via liver; inactivated by tissue; renal excreted.

Avoid in patients with GFR <50 mL/min (toxic metabolites accumulate).

Dosage should probably be adjusted in liver disease.

Supplemental dose suggested after HD.

Side Effects: Anorexia, nausea and vomiting, abdominal pain, diarrhea, acute or chronic pulmonary hypersensitivity reactions that can cause exertional dyspnea, malaise, altered pulmonary function tests, interstitial pneumonitis or fibrosis, hemolytic anemia, hepatitis.

Drug Interactions: Uricosuric agents can decrease its tubular secretion, causing higher serum levels and diminished efficacy.

Cautions: Contraindicated in anuria or oliguria and in pregnant patients at term (hemolytic anemia can occur secondary to G6PD deficiency).

Pearls: Cost $$$ (100 tablets retail: 50 mg ≈$65, 100 mg ≈$110).

Pregnancy category not established; *see* Cautions.

NITROGLYCERIN [IV] (NTG)

Dose: Initial, 5–20 μg/min; may increase in increments of 5–20 μg/min. Some physicians consider 400 μg/min the maximum dose, but this will vary from one institution to another.

Actions: Nitrate that relaxes vascular smooth muscle (venous>arterial) and dilates coronary arteries; used to treat angina.

Clearance: Catabolized in the liver.

Dosage adjustment probably not needed in impaired renal function.

Side Effects: Headache, hypotension, reflex tachycardia.

Pearls: Cost $ (≈$10/d wholesale).

Tolerance can develop.

Pregnancy category C.

NITROGLYCERIN paste (Nitrol 2% Ointment, Nitropaste)

Dose: Apply 1–2 inches topically q4–6h.

Side Effects: Headache (common), light-headedness, fainting, hypotension, nausea and vomiting, contact dermatitis.

Pearls: Cost $ (60 g ≈$10 wholesale).
Pregnancy category C.

NITROGLYCERIN patch (Minitran, Nitro-Dur, Transderm-Nitro)

Dose: *Note:* Prescribing basis for nitroglycerin patches has been changed from mg/d to mg/h.
Initial, 0.2–0.4 mg/h (approximately equivalent to 5–10 mg/d with former dosing system).

Preparations: New patch sizes: 0.1, 0.2, 0.3, 0.4, 0.5, and 0.6 mg/h.

Actions: Dermal patch that slowly releases nitroglycerin, which relaxes vascular smooth muscle (venous>arterial) and dilates coronary arteries; used to treat CAD.

Clearance: Metabolized via liver.
No change in dosage needed for impaired renal function.

Side Effects: Headache, light-headedness, fainting, hypotension, nausea and vomiting, dermatitis.

Pearls: Cost: generic $$, brands $$$ (30 patches retail: generic ≈$10, brands ≈$44).
Some authorities recommend removing patch at night to avoid development of tolerance.
Pregnancy category C.

NITROGLYCERIN spray (Nitrolingual)

Dose: Use dependent.
Angina prophylaxis: 0.4–0.8 mg (1 or 2 sprayed doses) under or on the tongue 5–10 min before activity.

Angina: 0.4–0.8 mg (1 or 2 sprayed doses) under or on the tongue; max, 3 doses within 15 min.

Preparations: 14.49 g metered-dose aerosol preparation that provides 200 doses.

NITROGLYCERIN sublingual tablets (Nitrostat)

Dose: Use dependent.
Angina prophylaxis: 1 tablet SL 5–10 min before activity.
Angina: 1 tablet SL q5min, up to 3 tablets if necessary.
Usual prescribed pill size is 1/150 grain; consider using 1/400 grain tablet in patients very sensitive to nitroglycerin.

Preparations: 1/100, 1/150, and 1/400 grain tablets.

Side Effects: Hypotension, headache.

Pearls: Cost $ (≈$6 retail/100 tablets).
Pills can lose their effectiveness over time; those still fresh enough to be effective will often "tingle" or "bubble" when placed underneath the tongue, while pills that have lost their effectiveness may not.
Pregnancy category C.

Nitrol: *see* NITROGLYCERIN paste

Nitrolingual: *see* NITROGLYCERIN spray

Nitropaste: *see* NITROGLYCERIN paste

NITROPRUSSIDE (Nipride)

Dose: 0.5–8.0 µg/kg/min.

Actions: Nitrate that relaxes vascular smooth muscle (arterial>venous), causing vasodilatation; used to treat hypertension and as afterload-reducing agent.

Clearance: Decomposed by nonenzymatic processes to cyanide, much of which is converted to thiocyanate by an enzyme located in the liver and kidneys.

One source recommends no change in dosage for impaired renal function; another source notes that risks of cyanide and thiocyanate toxicity are increased in renal or hepatic disease. Thus, it seems prudent to use nitroprusside with caution and to monitor thiocyanate levels in patients with renal or hepatic disease.

Side Effects: Hypotension, thiocyanate toxicity, rare cyanide toxicity (in severe liver dysfunction).

Pearls: Cost $$ ($\approx$$80/d wholesale).

Its toxic metabolite thiocyanate can cause seizure, coma, or hypothyroidism; thiocyanate levels <10 mg/dL are usually well tolerated, while levels >20 mg/dL are associated with increased toxicity.

Cyanide inhibits the cytochrome system, leading to inhibition of aerobic metabolism and increased lactate production; metabolic acidosis may be an early sign of cyanide toxicity.

Nitrostat: see NITROGLYCERIN sublingual tablets

NIZATIDINE (Axid)

Dose: Use dependent.
Active duodenal ulcer: 300 mg PO qhs or 150 mg PO bid.
Maintenance of healed duodenal ulcer: 150 mg PO qhs.

Preparations: 150 and 300 mg Axid Pulvules.

Actions: H_2-blocker; used to treat peptic ulcer disease.

Clearance: Moderately to markedly increase dosing interval in impaired renal function.

Side Effects: Decreased platelets, somnolence, sweating, urticaria, exfoliative dermatitis.

Drug Interactions: Can raise serum salicylate levels in patients taking high-dose aspirin.

Pearls: Cost $$$ ($1–$2/d retail).
Pregnancy category C.

Nizoral: see KETOCONAZOLE

Nizoral topical: see KETOCONAZOLE topical

Norcuron: see VECURONIUM

NOREPINEPHRINE (Levophed)

Dose: Most sources recommend an initial infusion rate of 8–12 μg/min for treatment of shock; some physicians will begin therapy for milder forms of hypotension with a lower infusion rate of 2–4 μg/min. In either case, dosage should be adjusted based on BP; required maintenance dose is usually 2–4 μg/min.

Actions: Strong α-adrenergic stimulator that increases peripheral vascular resistance (has minimal β-adrenergic stimulation); used to treat hypotension.

Side Effects: Tissue ischemia, decreased renal perfusion and urine output.

Cautions: Contraindicated in occlusive vascular disease.
  Use with extreme caution in patients taking MAOI or tricyclics (will substantially increase BP).

Pearls: Give through a large vein when possible.
  Give phentolamine if extravasated.
  May contain sulfite.
  Pregnancy category C.

NORETHINDRONE: see Norinyl, Ortho-Novum, Tri-Norinyl oral contraceptive pills

NORFLOXACIN (Noroxin)

Dose: 400 mg PO bid for 7–21 days, taken 1 h before or 2 h after meals.

Preparations: 400 mg tablets.

Actions: Synthetic bactericidal fluoroquinolone antibiotic that inhibits DNA synthesis; used to treat urinary tract infections, including *P. aeruginosa*, staph, strep, and enterococci.

Clearance: Metabolized via liver to active metabolites; biliary and renal excreted.

Moderately increase dosing interval in impaired renal function; avoid in ESRD.

Dosage adjustment probably not needed in patients with liver disease but good renal function.

Supplemental dose not required after HD.

Side Effects: Generally well tolerated.

Drug Interactions: Nitrofurantoin can antagonize its actions. Probenecid can decrease its urinary excretion. Concurrent use with antacids, sucralfate, or iron salts can decrease its absorption. Can potentiate effects of anticoagulants and increase theophylline toxicity and cyclosporine-induced nephrotoxicity.

Cautions: Contraindicated in patients <18 years old.

Should probably not be used in pregnant or potentially pregnant patients.

Pearls: Cost $$$ (generic ≈$37/wk); see under Penicillin for a comparison of weekly costs for brand-name and generic oral antibiotics.

Should *not* be used to treat systemic infections (does not achieve good serum levels).

Classified as pregnancy category C, but also noted to be contraindicated during pregnancy.

Norinyl oral contraceptive pills (NORETHINDRONE + ETHINYL ESTRADIOL or NORETHINDRONE + MESTRANOL)

Dose: 1 pill PO qd, preferably qhs; with 21-day regimen, take no pills on days 22–28 then begin a new cycle (3 weeks on, 1 week off).

Take first pill on the first Sunday after onset of menses, or that Sunday if it is first day of menses.

Preparations: Available in 21- and 28-pill preparations. Norinyl 1 + 35: 1 mg norethindrone and 0.035 mg ethinyl estradiol. Norinyl 1 + 50: 1 mg norethindrone and 0.050 mg mestranol.

Actions: Combination oral contraceptive; used to prevent pregnancy.

Side Effects: Serious vascular complications, menstrual changes, breakthrough bleeding, cervical and breast changes, vaginal candidiasis, hypertension, nausea and vomiting, liver tumors, GI distress, edema, weight changes, migraine headache, rash, depression, glucose intolerance, visual changes from alteration in corneal curvature, intolerance for contact lenses.

Drug Interactions: Contraceptive effectiveness can be decreased by antibiotics (ampicillin, chloramphenicol, isoniazid, nitrofurantoin, penicillin V, phenytoin, rifampin, sulfonamides, tetracycline), anxiolytics, phenylbutazones, barbiturates, antimigraine medications, analgesics, and tranquilizers.

Cautions: Contraindicated in patients with thromboembolic or thrombophlebitic disorders, cardiovascular or cerebrovascular disease, vaginal bleeding of unknown cause, endometrial or other estrogen-dependent tumors, known or suspected breast cancer, jaundice, hepatic tumors, or possible pregnancy.

Cigarette smoking increases risk of serious cardiovascular complications; patients should be *strongly* advised not to smoke.

Pearls: Cost $$$ ($\approx$$20/mo retail).

Patients should undergo complete workup prior to use, with special attention to history of abnormal vaginal bleeding, BP, breast examination, and pelvic examination including cervical cytology.

Pregnancy category X.

Normodyne: see LABETALOL

Noroxin: see NORFLOXACIN

Norpace: see DISOPYRAMIDE

Norplant: see LEVONORGESTREL

Norpramin: see DESIPRAMINE

NORTRIPTYLINE (Aventyl, Pamelor)

Dose: Usual, 25 mg PO tid–qid; max, 150 mg daily (maximum in elderly patients, 30–50 mg daily).

Preparations: Pamelor: 10, 25, 50, and 75 mg tablets; 16 oz bottles containing 10 mg/5 mL (1 tsp); Aventyl: 10 and 25 mg capsules; 16 oz bottles containing 10 mg/5 mL (1 tsp).

Actions: Tricyclic; used to treat depression.

Clearance: Metabolized via liver.
    No change in dosage needed for impaired renal function.
    One source suggests slightly reducing dosage in liver disease, though little data is available.
    Supplemental dose not required after HD or PD.

Side Effects: Prolonged conduction time, sinus tachycardia, tremors, diaphoresis.

Drug Interactions: Concomitant use with MAOI causes hyperpyretic crisis, convulsion, and death. Increases risk of arrhythmia in patients receiving thyroid replacement therapy.

Cautions: Contraindicated in patients who have taken MAOI within 2 weeks.
    Use with caution in cardiac disease, glaucoma, or urine retention (because of its anticholinergic and conduction effects).

Pearls: Cost $$$$ (25 mg Pamelor ≈$2.50/d retail); no generic form available.
    Consider monitoring serum level when dosage exceeds 100 mg daily.
    "Therapeutic window" is 50–150 µg/mL.
    Signs and symptoms of overdose include confusion, restlessness, agitation, vomiting, hyperpyrexia, muscle rigidity, hyperactive reflexes, tachycardia, ECG evidence of impaired conduction, ventricular arrhythmias, hypotension and shock, CHF, stupor, coma, seizures, and respiratory depression.
    Pregnancy category not established.

NTG: *see* **NITROGLYCERIN**

Nuprin: *see* **IBUPROFEN**

Nydriazid: *see* **ISONIAZID**

NYSTATIN (Mycostatin cream and ointment)

Dose: Apply to skin bid.

Preparations: 15 and 30 g cream and ointment; 15 g powder.

Actions: Topical antifungal; used to treat candidiasis.

OFLOXACIN (Floxin)

Dose: Disease dependent (as recommended by manufacturer). Should be taken at least 1/2h before or at least 2h after meals.

Lower respiratory tract infection: 400 mg PO q12h for 10 days.

Urinary tract infection: 200 mg PO q12h for 3 days for cystitis caused by *E. coli* or *K. pneumoniae,* 7 days for cystitis caused by other organisms, or 10 days for "complicated" urinary tract infections.

Prostatitis: 300 mg PO q12h for 6 weeks.

Acute, uncomplicated gonorrhea: Single dose of 400 mg PO.

Cervicitis/urethritis from *Chlamydia* [+/-] *N. gonorrhoeae:* 300 mg PO q12h for 7 days.

Mild to moderate infection of skin or skin structures: 400 mg PO q12h for 10 days.

Preparations: 200, 300, and 400 mg tablets.

Actions: Broad-spectrum fluoroquinolone that inhibits DNA gyrase. Good gram (+) coverage including *S. aureus* and MRSA (but *not* enterococci); excellent gram (−) coverage including *P. aeruginosa;* poor anaerobic coverage. Also covers *Chlamydia* (unlike Cipro) and has in vitro activity against atypical pneumonia pathogens (*Mycoplasma, Chlamydia pneumoniae* (TWAR), and *Legionella*).

Clearance: Primarily excreted unchanged in urine.

Adjust dosage in impaired renal function: for CrCl 10–50 mL/min, increase dosing interval to q24h; for CrCl <10 mL/min, give 1/2 recommended dose q24h.

Side Effects: Usually well tolerated. Rare side effects include nausea, diarrhea, GI distress, headache, and insomnia.

Drug Interactions: Raises serum level of theophylline. Concomitant use with sucralfate, iron, multivitamins containing zinc, or antacids containing calcium, magnesium, or aluminum can subtantially decrease its absorption.

Cautions: Do not use in patients <18 years old.

Pearls: Cost $$$ (≈$53/wk of therapy); see under Penicillin for a comparison of weekly costs for brand-name and generic oral antibiotics.

Avoid excessive exposure to sunlight (similar drugs have been associated with increased photosensitivity).

Pregnancy category C.

OLSALAZINE SODIUM (Dipentum)

Dose: 500 mg PO bid with food.

Preparations: 250 mg capsules.

Actions: Salicylate compound that delivers 5-ASA to the colon; used in maintenance therapy for ulcerative colitis in patients who do not tolerate sulfasalazine (Azulfidine).

Clearance: Only about 2.4% is absorbed; the rest remains in the GI tract.

Side Effects: Diarrhea, abdominal cramps or pain, nausea.

Pearls: Cost $$$$ (≈$2/d retail); sulfasalazine costs ≈$0.50/d retail.

Unlike sulfasalazine, does not have a sulfa-containing sulfapyridine component and so is better tolerated in patients allergic or sensitive to sulfa.

Pregnancy category C.

OMEPRAZOLE (Prilosec; formerly Losec)

Dose: 20 mg PO qd for 4–8 weeks, taken before meals.

Preparations: 20 mg capsules.

Actions: Medication that inhibits H^+/K^+-ATPase of gastric parietal cells, inhibiting the proton pump; used to treat peptic ulcer disease and severe esophageal reflux.

Side Effects: Minimal reported common side effects.

Drug Interactions: Prolongs elimination of diazepam, warfarin, phenytoin, and other drugs that are oxidized in the liver.

Pearls: Cost $$$$ ($\approx$$3/tablet retail).
 Can interfere with drugs absorbed at acid gastric pH (ketoconazole, ampicillin, iron salts, etc.).
 Renamed Prilosec, possibly to avoid confusion with "Lasix."
 Pregnancy category C.

ONDANSETRON (Zofran)

Dose: 0.15 mg/kg IV over 15 min, given 30 min before chemotherapy and repeated 4 and 8 h later (total of three 0.15 mg/kg doses).

Actions: Selective serotonin receptor antagonist; used to prevent chemotherapy-induced nausea and vomiting.

Clearance: Extensively metabolized in liver by cytochrome P-450. Clearance is reduced and $t_{1/2}$ prolonged in patients >75 years old.

Side Effects: Headache, dizziness, diarrhea, constipation, elevated LFTs, extrapyramidal effects.

Drug Interactions: Can affect other serotonin-mediated medications (buspirone, fluoxetine, cyproheptadine, clomipramine).

Pearls: Cost $$$$ (40 mg vial $200).
 Pregnancy category B.

Opticrom: see CROMOLYN SODIUM

Organidin (IODINATED GLYCEROL)

Dose: Delivery dependent.
  PO: 2 tablets given with liquid qid.
  Solution: 20 drops PO qid.
  Elixir: 1 tsp PO qid.

Preparations: 30 mg tablets; 30 mL dropper bottles of solution; 1 pint and 1 gallon bottles of elixir.

Actions: Mucolytic-expectorant that increases output of respiratory tract fluid and helps to liquefy tenacious mucus in the bronchial tree; used to treat nonproductive cough secondary to pulmonary infection.

Side Effects: Rash, hypersensitivity reactions, rare GI discomfort, hypothyroidism.

Cautions: Contraindicated in pregnant or potentially pregnant patients and in patients with history of hypersensitivity to iodides. Use with caution in patients with history of thyroid disease.

Pearls: Cost $ (PO ≈$1/d wholesale).
  Actual clinical benefits are controversial.
  Pregnancy category X.

Orinase: see TOLBUTAMIDE

Ortho-Novum contraceptive pills (NORETHINDRONE + ETHINYL ESTRADIOL or NORETHINDRONE + MESTRANOL)

Dose: 1 tablet PO qd; with 21-day regimen, take no pills on days 22–28 then begin a new cycle (3 weeks on, 1 week off).
  For 21-pill preparations of Ortho-Novum 7/7/7 or 10/11 and for all 28-pill preparations, take first tablet on the first Sunday after onset of menses, or that Sunday if it is first day of menses; for 21-pill preparations of Ortho-Novum 1/35 or 1/50, take first tablet on the fifth day of the menstrual cycle, counting the first day of menses as day 1.

Preparations: Available in 21- and 28-tablet preparations; last 7 tablets in 28-tablet preparation usually contain only inert ingredients. Quantities of norethindrone (N), ethinyl estradiol (E), and mestranol (N) in the various preparations: Ortho-Novum 7/7/7: first week, 0.5 mg N and 0.035 mg E; second week, 0.75 mg N and 0.035 mg E; third week, 1.0 mg N and 0.035 mg E. Ortho-Novum 1/35: fixed dose of 1 mg N and 0.035 mg E. Ortho-Novum 1/50: fixed dose of 1 mg N and 0.050 mg M. Ortho-Novum 10/11: first 10 days, 0.5 mg N and 0.035 mg E; days 11–21, 1.0 mg N and 0.035 mg E.

Actions: Combination oral contraceptive; used to prevent pregnancy.

Side Effects: Serious vascular complications, menstrual changes, hypertension, gallbladder disease, liver tumors, nausea and vomiting, GI distress, breakthrough bleeding, edema, breast changes, weight changes, cervical changes, migraine headache, rash, depression, glucose intolerance, vaginal candidiasis, visual changes from alteration in corneal curvature, intolerance for contact lenses.

Drug Interactions: Contraceptive effectiveness can be decreased by antibiotics (ampicillin, chloramphenicol, isoniazid, nitrofurantoin, penicillin V, rifampin, sulfonamides, tetracycline), analgesics, anxiolytics, antimigraine agents, barbiturates, and phenylbutazone.

Cautions: Contraindicated in patients with thromboembolic or thrombophlebitic disorders, cardiovascular or cerebrovascular disease, vaginal bleeding of unknown cause, endometrial or other estrogen-dependent neoplasms, known or suspected breast cancer, cholestatic jaundice or jaundice with prior pill use, hepatic adenoma or carcinoma, or known or suspected pregnancy.

Cigarette smoking increases risk of serious cardiovascular complications; patients should be *strongly* advised not to smoke.

Pearls: Cost $$$ ($\approx$$20/mo retail).

Patients should undergo complete workup prior to use with special attention to history of abnormal vaginal bleeding, BP, breast examination, and pelvic examination including cervical cytology.

Pregnancy category X.

Os-Cal: see CALCIUM CARBONATE

OXACILLIN

Dose: 1–2 g IM or IV q4–6h.

Actions: Bactericidal β-lactamase–resistant penicillin that inhibits cell wall synthesis. Excellent gram (+) coverage including staph and strep (but *not* MSRA or enterococci); no gram (−) coverage; poor anaerobic coverage.

Clearance: Metabolized via liver; renal excreted.
No change in dosage needed for impaired renal function.
Avoid in liver disease (because of hepatotoxicity).
Supplemental dose not required after HD or PD.

Side Effects: Rash, occasional elevated LFTs, hepatitis and jaundice, interstitial nephritis, rare neutropenia.

Cautions: Contraindicated in patients with penicillin allergy.

Pearls: Cost $$$ (≈$60/d wholesale).
Monitor LFTs during prolonged therapy.
Contains high Na^+ load.
Penicillin provides better coverage than oxacillin for strep.
Pregnancy category C.

OXAZEPAM (Serax)

Dose: 10–30 mg PO tid–qid.

Preparations: 10, 15, and 30 mg capsules.

Actions: Short-acting benzodiazepine with sedative and anxiolytic effects; used to treat anxiety.

Clearance: Metabolized via liver.
No change in dosage recommended for impaired renal function; can cause excess sedation or encephalopathy in ESRD.
No change in dosage needed for liver disease.
Supplemental dose not required after HD.

Side Effects: Transient mild drowsiness, rare decreased WBCs and liver dysfunction, rare but significant hypotension.

Drug Interactions: Potentiates CNS depressant effects of other CNS depressants.

Cautions: Should probably not be used by pregnant or potentially pregnant patients.

Pearls: Cost: generic $$$, Serax $$$$ (100 tablets retail: 15 mg generic ≈$30, 15 mg Serax ≈$70, 30 mg generic ≈$45, 30 mg Serax ≈$100).

Abrupt discontinuance after extended use can precipitate barbiturate-like withdrawal reaction.

Is particularly useful in elderly patients.

Has relatively short $t_{1/2}$.

Periodically check CBC and LFTs.

Oxazepam has not been adequately studied, but other minor anxiolytics *are* associated with congenital malformations when taken during pregnancy.

Oxy-5, Oxy-10: see BENZOYL PEROXIDE

OXYBUTYNIN (Ditropan)

Dose: 5 mg or 5 mL (1 tsp) PO bid–qid.

Preparations: 5 mg tablets; 16 oz bottles of syrup containing 5 mg/5 mL (1 tsp).

Actions: Urinary antispasmodic; used to treat urinary frequency and incontinence secondary to neurogenic bladder.

Clearance: Metabolized via liver.

Side Effects: Dizziness, drowsiness, insomnia, dry mouth, tachycardia, palpitations, constipation, urinary hesitancy and retention, impotence, hallucinations, elevated intraocular pressure.

Drug Interactions: Raises serum level of digoxin. Increases anticholinergic blockade.

Cautions: Contraindicated in patients with elevated intraocular pressure associated with angle-closure glaucoma, any disease associated with reduced intestinal motility, or myasthenia gravis.

Use with caution in elderly patients and in patients with hepatic disease, renal disease, or autonomic neuropathy.

Pearls: Cost: generic $$, Ditropan $$$ (generic ≈$0.75/d retail, Ditropan ≈$1.30/d retail).
Pregnancy category B.

OXYCODONE: see Percocet, Percodan

OXYMETAZOLINE (Afrin)

Dose: 2–4 drops (written "gtt") or sprays of 0.05% solution intranasally bid.

Actions: Long-acting α-adrenergic agonist that causes local vasoconstriction; used to treat nasal congestion.

Side Effects: Rebound nasal congestion or irritation with long-term use, hypotension or hypertension, headache, insomnia.

Pearls: Cost $.
Some physicians use intranasal steroids to treat rebound nasal congestion.
Pregnancy category not established.

Pamelor: see NORTRIPTYLINE

Pancrease: see PANCRELIPASE

PANCRELIPASE (Pancrease, Viokase)

Dose: 1–3 capsules (Pancrease) or 1–3 tablets (Viokase) with each meal and 1 capsule with snacks.

Preparations: Capsules containing lipase, protease, and amylase.

Side Effects: GI discomfort, rare allergic-type reactions.

Pearls: Cost $$$$ (≈$2/d retail).
Pregnancy category D.

PANCURONIUM (Pavulon)

Dose: Initially give 0.04–0.10 mg/kg IV push; maintenance, 0.01–0.02 mg/kg IV push given q20–60min as required.

Preparations: 10 mL vials containing 1 mg/mL; 2 and 5 mL ampules containing 2 mg/mL.

Actions: Neuromuscular blocking agent that relaxes skeletal muscle; used to induce paralysis during intubation, status epilepticus, and other clinical situations.

Clearance: Metabolized via liver; renal excreted.

$t_{1/2}$ is increased in liver dysfunction and in impaired renal function.

No change in dosage needed for impaired renal function; avoid if GFR <10 mL/min.

Side Effects: Tachycardia (from acetylcholine block), slight elevation in BP.

Pearls: Cost $ (10 mg ≈$13 wholesale).

Pregnancy category C.

Paraplatin:see CARBOPLATIN

Parlodel: see BROMOCRIPTINE MESYLATE

Pavulon: see PANCURONIUM

PCE 333, 500: see ERYTHROMYCIN

PENICILLIN (Pen-Vee K)

Dose: Infection dependent and variable by source. Possible regimens include:

Strep throat: Penicillin VK 250 mg PO qid for 10 days, taken 30 min before or 2 h after meals.

Pneumococcal pneumonia: Procaine penicillin G 600,000 units IV q6h; may switch to penicillin VK 250 mg PO qid.

Aspiration pneumonia: Procaine penicillin G 2,000,000 units IV q4h.

S. pneumoniae or *N. meningitidis* meningitis: Procaine penicillin G 2,000,000 units IV q2h.

Endocarditis prophylaxis: Penicillin V 2 g PO 1 h before procedure and 1 g PO 6 h later.

Pediatric dose: Children <12 years old, 15–50 mg/kg PO daily in 3 or 4 divided doses; children ≥12 years, same as adult dose.

Preparations: 125, 250, and 500 mg tablets of penicillin V (Pen-Vee K, etc.); various concentrations of penicillin G for injection.

Actions: Bactericidal antibiotic that inhibits cell wall synthesis. Good gram (+) coverage including enterococci (but *not* staph); limited gram (−) coverage (but *not* β-lactamase–producing organisms); good anaerobic coverage (but *not* some *Bacteroides*.)

Clearance: Some liver metabolism; primarily renal excreted.
Moderately reduce dosage in impaired renal function.
No change in dosage needed for liver disease.
Supplemental dose suggested after HD or PD.

Side Effects: PO: nausea and vomiting, epigastric distress, diarrhea, and black, hairy tongue.

PO or IV: hypersensitivity reactions (rash, exfoliative dermatitis, urticaria), serum sickness (fever, chills, edema, arthralgia, prostration), anaphylactic reaction, interstitial nephritis, drug fever, rare hemolytic anemia, reduced WBCs and platelets, neuropathy or neurotoxicity.

Drug Interactions: Possible drug antagonism with chloramphenicol and tetracycline. Decreases contraceptive effect of some oral contraceptives. Uricosurics (probenecid, indomethacin, etc.) can raise its serum level.

Cautions: Contraindicated in patients with penicillin allergy.

Pearls: Cost \$ (IV ≈\$1 wholesale/1,000,000 units, \$4–\$12/d wholesale); markedly less expensive than many other IV antibiotics.

Give penicillin G PO 30 min before or 2 h after meals (to assure maximum absorption); may give penicillin VK with meals.

Pregnancy category not established.

Cost Comparison

Average retail cost for 1 week of PO therapy with brand-name and generic drugs:

AMOX	$ 8	Ceclor	$59	Floxin	$53
AMP	$ 7	Ceftin	$45	Keflex	$37
Augment	$49	Cipro	$43	Keftab	$32
Bactrim	$20	DICLOX	$20	NORFLOX	$37
Biaxin	$43	ERYTHRO	$10	PCN VK	$ 6

Pentam: see PENTAMIDINE

PENTAMIDINE (NebuPent, Pentam)

Dose: Use dependent.
PCP prevention: 300 mg by Respigard nebulizer monthly.
Acute therapy: 4 mg/kg/d IV for 14 days.

Preparations: Pentam: 300 mg vials to be diluted for injection; Nebupent: 300 mg vials to be diluted for delivery by nebulizer.

Actions: Antiprotozoal agent that interferes with folate transmission; used to treat PCP.

Clearance: Primarily cleared by nonrenal mechanisms.
Slightly increase dosing interval in impaired renal function.
Not removed by dialysis.

Side Effects: Inhaled: cough and bronchospasm.
IV, reduced WBCs and platelets, increased creatinine, elevated LFTs, hypotension, hypoglycemia, hyperglycemia, pancreatitis, fever, cardiac arrhythmia.
May be associated with fatigue, bitter or metallic taste, shortness of breath, anorexia, dizziness, rash, nausea and vomiting, pharyngitis, chest pain or congestion, night sweats or chills. Rare deaths have been reported secondary to hypotension, hypoglycemia, or cardiac arrhythmias.

Pearls: Cost $$$$ (2-week IV course $1800 wholesale).
Patients on PCP prophylaxis can *still* develop PCP.
Follow CBC, glucose, LFTs, BUN, creatinine, and ECG.

Preventive therapy is indicated in high-risk patients (T_4 count <200 or previous PCP infection).
Pregnancy category C.

PENTOBARBITAL (Nembutal)

Dose: 3–5 mg/kg IV loading dose; maintenance, 2–3.5 mg/kg IV given hourly prn.

Preparations: 2 mL vials containing 50 mg/mL.

Actions: Barbiturate; used to treat convulsions and to induce coma.

Clearance: Metabolized via liver.
  Reduce dosage in liver disease.

Drug Interactions: Induces hepatic enzymes.

Cautions: Can cause respiratory depression and hypotension.

Pearls: Cost $ (100 mg ≈$2 wholesale).
  Avoid perivascular extravasation.
  Pregnancy category D.

PENTOXIFYLLINE (Trental)

Dose: Usual, 400 mg PO tid with meals; may reduce dosage to 400 mg PO bid if GI or CNS side effects occur.

Preparations: 400 mg controlled-release tablets.

Actions: Methyl xanthine analog that may act by reducing blood viscosity, improving RBC flexibility, reducing RBC and platelet aggregation, and decreasing elevated plasma fibrinogen; used to treat intermittent claudication from peripheral vascular disease.

Clearance: Metabolized via liver.
  No change in dosage needed for impaired renal function.

Side Effects: Rare side effects include nausea and vomiting and CNS symptoms.

Pearls: Cost $$$ (≈$1.20/d retail); no generic form available.

Can cause a further small reduction in BP in patients taking antihypertensive agents.

Bleeding and increased PT have been reported in patients both taking and not taking warfarin or antiplatelet agents, but a causal relationship has not been clearly shown; consider more frequent PT monitoring in patients taking warfarin.

Pregnancy category C.

Pen-Vee K: see PENICILLIN

Pepcid: see FAMOTIDINE

Percocet (OXYCODONE + ACETAMINOPHEN)

Dose: 1 tablet PO q6h prn.

Preparations: Each tablet contains 5 mg oxycodone and 325 mg acetaminophen.

Actions: Narcotic analgesic with antipyretic actions; used to treat moderate to moderately severe pain.

Clearance: Little information available; probably metabolized via liver with some renal excretion of active metabolites.

Dosing interval should probably be increased in liver disease.

Side Effects: Light-headedness, dizziness, sedation, nausea and vomiting, constipation, elevated CSF pressure, euphoria.

Cautions: Contraindicated in patients with CNS injury or lesions.

Use with caution in elderly or debilitated patients and in patients with severely impaired hepatic or renal function, hypothyroidism, Addison's disease, prostate hypertrophy, or urethral stricture.

Pearls: Cost: generic $$, Percocet $$$ (100 tablets retail: generic ≈$22, Percocet ≈$65).

Raises serum levels of amylase and lipase.

Can produce drug dependency.

Pregnancy category C.

Percodan (OXYCODONE HCL, OXYCODONE TEREPHTHALATE + ASA)

Dose: 1 tablet PO q6h prn.

Preparations: Each tablet contains 4.5 mg oxycodone HCl, 0.38 mg oxycodone terephthalate, and 325 mg ASA.

Actions: Narcotic analgesic with salicylate antipyretic action; used to treat moderate to moderately severe pain.

Clearance: Little information available; oxycodone is probably liver metabolized with some renal excretion of active metabolites.
   Dosing interval should probably be increased in liver disease.

Side Effects: Light-headedness, dizziness, sedation, nausea and vomiting, gastric irritation, upper GI bleeding, constipation, rash, pruritus, elevated CSF pressure.

Cautions: Contraindicated in patients with CNS injury or lesions or with ASA allergy.
   Use with caution in elderly or debilitated patients and in patients with severely impaired hepatic or renal function, hypothyroidism, Addison's disease, prostate hypertrophy, urethral stricture, or history of peptic ulcer disease or upper GI bleeding.

Pearls: Cost: generic $$, Percodan $$$ (100 tablets retail: generic ≈$20, Percodan $67).
   Can produce drug dependency.
   Pregnancy category not established.

Periactin: see CYPROHEPTADINE

Peri-Colace (CASANTHRANOL + DOCUSATE)

Dose: 1 or 2 capsules prn–bid, depending on need and use.

Preparations: Each capsule contains 30 mg casanthranol and 100 mg docusate (Colace).

Actions: Combination mild stimulant laxative and stool softener that provides gently peristaltic stimulation and helps to keep stools softer for easier passage.

Side Effects: Rare GI discomfort.

Pearls: Cost $$ (100 tablets retail: generic $14, PeriColace ≈$27).

Usually induces bowel movement overnight or in 8–12 h.

Should be taken with generous amount of fluid.

PERPHENAZINE (Trilafon, etc.)

Dose: Disease and delivery dependent.

Nausea and vomiting: PO, 6–16 mg daily in divided doses (suggestions for each dose range from 2–8 mg); IV: 5 mg q6h prn; IM: 5–10 mg.

Acute psychosis: 5–10 mg IM or IV.

Preparations: 2, 4, 8, and 16 mg tablets; 4 oz bottle with graduated dropper containing 16 mg/5 mL (1 tsp); 1 mL ampules containing 5 mg/mL for injection.

Actions: Phenothiazine that acts at all levels of the nervous system; used to treat severe nausea and vomiting and psychotic disorders.

Clearance: Primary mechanism of clearance is most likely liver metabolism.

Manufacturer suggests using with caution in renal disease.

Supplemental dose not required after dialysis.

Side Effects: Orthostatic hypotension, elevated LFTs and cholestatic jaundice, impairment of mental and physical abilities, fever, anticholinergic effects (dry mouth, blurred vision, urine retention, etc.), drowsiness, extrapyramidal reactions, tardive dyskinesia, neuroleptic malignant syndrome.

Drug Interactions: Anatacids reduce its absorption. Barbiturates can decrease its effectiveness. Potentiates CNS depressant effects of other CNS depressants. Can raise serum levels of antidepressants.

Cautions: Contraindicated in patients with liver damage, blood dyscrasias, bone marrow depression, subcortical brain damage, or depressed consciousness and in patients taking large doses of other CNS depressants.

Use with caution in elderly patients.

Pearls: Cost $$ (IV ≈$15/d wholesale).
Follow CBC, LFTs, and renal function.
Pregnancy category not established.

Persantine: see DIPYRIDAMOLE

Phazyme: see SIMETHICONE

PHENAZOPYRIDINE (Pyridium)

Dose: 200 mg PO tid after meals.

Preparations: 100 and 200 mg tablets.

Actions: Excreted in urine, where its analgesic action relieves urinary pain, burning, urgency, and frequency.

Side Effects: Headache, rash, GI disturbances, staining of contact lenses, renal and hepatic toxicity (usually at overdose levels), hemolytic anemia, methemoglobinemia.

Pearls: Cost $$ (≈$0.40/d retail).
Pregnancy category B.

Phenergan: see PROMETHAZINE

PHENIRAMINE: see Naphcon-A ophthalmic solution

PHENOBARBITAL

Dose: Situation and disease dependent.
Initial therapy for status epilepticus: Recommendations for loading rate and initial IV dose vary significantly. Some sources recommend an injection rate of 60–100 mg/min; other sources note that injection at rates >60 mg/min can cause hypotension, severely reduced respirations and apnea, and laryngospasm. Initial dosage recommendations vary from 200–320 mg to 10 mg/kg IV.

Maximum dose is usually given as 20 mg/kg (patients can get respiratory depression and require intubation at this point).

Because suggested regimens vary so widely among sources, it is difficult to make any definitive recommendation for dosing. A possible initial regimen for status epilepticus that conforms with many sources would be 5 mg/kg IV given over 10 min. This dose may be repeated, if needed, after 30–60 min.

Chronic therapy for seizures: 100–300 mg PO qd.

Sedation: 30–120 mg daily given in 2 or 3 divided doses.

Preparations: 8, 15, 16, 30, 32, 60, 65, and 100 mg tablets; 20 mg/5 mL (1 tsp) elixir; 30, 60, 65, and 130 mg/mL injection.

Actions: Anticonvulsant, sedative.

Clearance: 50–75% liver metabolized; 25–50% renal excreted.

Slightly increase dosing interval in ESRD; no change needed for milder renal impairment.

Reduce dosage in liver dysfunction.

Renal excretion is increased with alkaline diuresis.

Supplemental dose suggested after HD or PD.

Side Effects: Severe allergic reactions, numerous CNS effects, nausea and vomiting, constipation, decreased WBC, decreased platelets, decreased hematocrit, bradycardia, hypotension, syncope.

Drug Interactions: Decreases PT in patients taking warfarin. Reduces effectiveness of digoxin and steroids.

Cautions: Contraindicated in patients with severe pulmonary insufficiency, sensitivity to barbiturates, or history of porphyria.

Pearls: Cost $ (≈$5 retail/100 tablets).

Therapeutic level varies depending on source and institution but is usually in the range of 10–40 μg/mL.

After IV dose, can take 15–30 min for peak level to be attained in the brain.

Withdrawal reactions can occur.

Intermittently check CBC in patients on chronic therapy.

Signs and symptoms of overdose include CNS depression, Cheyne-Stokes respiration, absent reflexes, severely depressed BP and temperature, and markedly increased HR.

Pregnancy category D.

PHENYLEPHRINE (Neo-Synephrine)

Dose: 1 or 2 drops (written "gtt") or sprays into each nostril q4h.

Actions: Topical decongestant that causes vasoconstriction through its α-agonist activity; used to treat nasal congestion.

Side Effects: Local irritation, rebound congestion.

Cautions: May be contraindicated in patients taking MAOI or tricyclics if systemically absorbed.
Relatively contraindicated in hypertension, hyperthyroidism, diabetes, and benign prostatic hypertrophy.

Pearls: Can antagonize antihypertensive agents if absorbed.

PHENYLEPHRINE eye drops

Dose: Use dependent.
Funduscopic examination: Instill 1 drop of 2.5% solution in the eye.
Uveitis: Instill 2.5% solution bid–tid.

Preparations: 2.5 and 10% solution (the 10% solution is rarely used).

Actions: Mydriatic with sympathomimetic properties; used to dilate the pupil.

Cautions: Use with caution in cardiovascular disease.

PHENYLPROPANOLAMINE (Acutrim; see also Allerest, Contac, Robitussin-CF)

Dose: For appetite suppression, 75 mg PO after breakfast.

Preparations: 75 mg tablets.

Actions: α-Agonist sympathomimetic; used as appetite suppressant, for stress incontinence in women, and in many over-the-counter cold products.

Clearance: Primarily excreted unchanged in urine.
Avoid in renal dysfunction.

Side Effects: Worsening of hypertension, restlessness, insomnia, agitation.

Drug Interactions: Concomitant use with MAOI, guanethidine, or indomethacin can precipitate hypertensive crisis.

Cautions: Contraindicated in significant cardiovascular disease or hypertension, hyperthyroidism, significant renal disease, and acute narrow-angle glaucoma.

Pearls: Used as decongestant in many cold preparations, including Allerest, Contac, and many others not listed in this guide.

PHENYTOIN (Dilantin)

Dose: Delivery dependent.
IV loading dose: 15–20 mg/kg (maximum rate, 50 mg/min; monitor ECG and BP).
PO loading dose: 1 g over 4 h, given as 400 mg initially, then 300 mg 2 h later, then another 300 mg 2 h later.
Usual maintenance: 100 mg PO tid–qid or 300–400 mg PO qd.

Preparations: 30, 50, and 100 mg tablets; 50 mg chewable tablets; 8 oz bottles of orange-vanilla flavored suspension containing 125 mg/5 mL (1 tsp); IV formulations for injection.

Actions: Medication used as (1) anticonvulsant, (2) antiarrhythmic, primarily for ventricular arrhythmias and certain atrial arrhythmias (particularly those secondary to digoxin toxicity).

Clearance: Metabolized via liver.
No change in dosage needed for impaired renal function.
Dosage may need to be reduced in severe liver disease, but dosing is probably best done by following serum drug levels.
Supplemental dose not required after HD or PD.

Side Effects (acute): Nausea and vomiting, rash, Stevens-Johnson syndrome, SLE, polyarteritis nodosa (PAN), elevated LFTs, reduced CBC, generalized lymphadenopathy, blood dyscrasias. Can cause increases in glucose, alkaline phosphatase, and GGTP, acne-like dermatitis, hirsuitism, and gingival hyperplasia.

Drug Interactions: Reduces efficacy of steroids, warfarin, quinidine, digoxin, and furosemide. Acute alcohol ingestion, ASA, cimetidine, and isoniazid raise its serum level. Chronic alcohol ingestion and antacids containing calcium reduce its serum level. Sucralfate reduces its intestinal absorption. In different patients, phenobarbital and valproic acid can either elevate or depress phenytoin levels, and phenytoin can either elevate or depress phenobarbital and valproic acid levels.

Pearls: Cost $$ ($\approx$$0.50/d retail).

Usual therapeutic level is 10–20 μg/mL.

In patients with significant renal failure, follow level of *free dilantin* secondary to reduced protein binding (therapeutic level of free dilantin is 1–2 μg/mL).

Abrupt withdrawal can precipitate seizure.

Acute alcohol ingestion can raise its serum level and chronic ingestion can reduce it.

Signs and symptoms of toxicity include delirium, psychosis, encephalopathy, cerebellar dysfunction, nystagmus, lethargy, and tremor.

Pregnancy category not established; is associated with increased congenital defects, which must be weighed against risk of seizing during pregnancy.

Phosphaljel: see ALUMINUM PHOSPHATE

Phospholine Iodide (ECHOTHIOPHATE IODIDE)

Dose: Instill 1 drop of 0.03–0.125% solution into the conjunctival sac qd–bid.

Actions: Cholinesterase-inhibiting eye drop; used to treat open-angle glaucoma.

Pearls: Pregnancy category C.

PHOSPHORUS (K-Phos, Neutra-Phos)

Dose: Brand dependent.

K-Phos: 1 or 2 tablets PO qid with full glass of water.

Neutra-Phos: 2 tablets PO bid–qid.

Preparations: 250 mg tablets of K-Phos Neutral; 250 mg tablets of Neutra-Phos.

Actions: Phosphorus supplement.

Side Effects: Diarrhea, GI upset, hypocalcemia.

Cautions: Use with caution in patients with renal compromise, cirrhosis, or CHF.

Pearls: Cost $$ ($\approx$$0.60/d retail).

IV phosphorus should be used cautiously and only for severe hypophosphatemia (serum phosphorus <1.0).

Signs and symptoms of severe hypophosphatemia include neuro-muscular effects (weakness, paresthesias, rhabdomyolysis, etc.), hematologic abnormalities (hemolysis, platelet dysfunction), and cardiac failure.

Pregnancy category C.

Pilocar: see PILOCARPINE

PILOCARPINE (Adsorbocarpine, Isopto Carpine, Pilocar, Pilopine)

Dose: Preparation dependent.

Solution: 1 or 2 drops (written "gtt") bid–qid.

Gel: 1/2-inch ribbon instilled into the lower conjunctival sac qhs or more frequently if needed.

Preparations: 4% gel of Pilopine HS; 1%, 4%, and many other preparations of solution.

Actions: Cholinergic miotic agent that increases outflow of aqueous humor; used to treat open-angle glaucoma.

Side Effects (local): Miosis and reduced night vision, burning, irritation, fluctuating refractive error (from ciliary muscle contraction), painful ciliary muscle spasm in younger patients.

Side Effects (systemic): Rare, but can include systemic cholinergic responses, cough, rhinorrhea, increased bronchial secretions, diarrhea, painful GI spasm, or anorexia.

Pearls: Solution usually must be given qid for consistent lowering of intraocular pressure.

Pilopine: see PILOCARPINE

PINDOLOL (Visken)

Dose: Initial, 5 mg PO bid; max, 60 mg PO daily.

Preparations: 5 and 10 mg tablets.

Actions: Nonselective β-blocker with intrinsic sympathomimetic activity; used to treat hypertension and CAD.

Clearance: Metabolized via liver; renal excreted.

No change in dosage needed for patients with impaired renal function but good liver function.

Reduce dosage in liver disease, especially in patients with both liver and renal disease.

Side Effects: Elevated LFTs, (rare) anxiety, lethargy, visual changes, bradycardia, claudication, hypotension, syncope.

Cautions: Contraindicated in bronchial asthma, second- or third-degree heart block, severe bradycardia, or cardiogenic shock.

Pearls: Cost $$$ (10 mg tablet ≈$0.80 retail).

Can get rebound effect with abrupt discontinuance.

May be a better β-blocking agent to use in patients with resting bradycardia or borderline CHF (because of its intrinsic sympathomimetic activity).

Has less cardioprotective effect than other β-blockers.

Taper when discontinuing (to avoid rebound reactions).

Pregnancy category B.

PIPERACILLIN

Dose: 3–4 g IV q4–6h. For less severe infections, may give up to 2 g IM per injection site.

Actions: Bactericidal semisynthetic antipseudomonal penicillin that inhibits cell wall synthesis. Good gram (+) coverage including enterococci and strep (but *not* staph); excellent gram (−) coverage including *P. aeruginosa;* good anaerobic coverage including *B. fragilis.*

Clearance: Renal excreted.
Slightly increase dosing interval in impaired renal function.
Sources differ on whether dosage should be reduced in liver dysfunction.
Supplemental dose suggested after HD.

Side Effects: Local thrombophlebitis, diarrhea, elevated LFTs, rash, eosinophilia, hypokalemia, neutropenia, anaphylactoid reaction.

Cautions: Contraindicated in patients with penicillin allergy.

Pearls: Cost $$$ (≈$100/d wholesale).
(+) CSF penetration in meningeal inflammation.
Can increase bleeding tendency in renal failure.
Pregnancy category B.

PIROXICAM (Feldene)

Dose: 20 mg PO qd or 10 mg PO bid.

Preparations: 10 and 20 mg tablets.

Actions: Nonsteroidal anti-inflammatory agent with analgesic and antipyretic actions; used to treat pain and inflammation.

Clearance: Metabolized via liver.
No change in dosage needed for impaired renal function.

Side Effects: GI irritation, peptic ulcer disease and upper GI bleeding, proteinuria, interstitial nephritis, nephrotic syndrome, worsening of "prerenal" renal failure, reversible platelet inhibition and increased bleeding time, edema.

Cautions: Contraindicated in patients with salicylate sensitivity or history of upper GI bleeding.
Should not be used in pregnant or potentially pregnant patients.

Pearls: Cost $$$$ ($\approx$\$2/d retail).
Has longest $t_{1/2}$ of the NSAIDs.
Not recommended for use during pregnancy.

Pitressin; *see* **VASOPRESSIN**

Plendil: *see* **FELODIPINE**

POLYETHYLENE GLYCOL; *see* **GoLYTELY**

POLYMYXIN B: *see* **Cortisporin, Neosporin**

POTASSIUM CHLORIDE (K-Dur, K-Tab, Micro-K, Slow-K)

Dose: 20–100 meq PO daily. Usually no more than 20–40 meq is given in a single dose.

Preparations: 10 meq tablets of K-Dur 10; 20 meq tablets of K-Dur 20; 10 meq tablets of K-Tab; 10 meq tablets of Micro-K; 8 meq tablets of Slow-K.

Actions: Potassium supplement.

Side Effects: GI irritation, hyperkalemia.

Cautions: Use with caution in renal failure and in patients taking K^+-sparing diuretics or ACE inhibitors.

Pearls: Cost $$$ (100 tablets retail: 10 meq generic $\approx$\$11; 20 meq K-Dur $\approx$\$40, 10 meq K-Tab $\approx$\$25, 10 meq Micro-K $\approx$\$16, 8 meq Slow-K $\approx$\$16).
K^+ depletion sufficient to cause hypokalemia usually requires loss of >200 meq of K^+ from total body stores.
Pregnancy category C.

Pravachol: *see* **PRAVASTATIN**

PRAVASTATIN (Pravachol)

Dose: Initial, 10–20 mg PO qhs; maintenance, 10–40 mg PO qhs.

Preparations: 10 and 20 mg tablets.

Actions: HMG-CoA reductase inhibitor that increases HDL and reduces total cholesterol and LDL; used to treat hyperlipidemia.

Clearance: Significant first-pass metabolism and elimination in feces; minor urinary excretion.
Dosage should be adjusted in liver disease or renal dysfunction.

Side Effects: Rare headache, weakness or fatigue, elevated LFTs, rare increased CPK, myositis, rhabdomyolysis.

Drug Interactions: Cholestyramine and colestipol can inhibit its absorption (give pravastatin at least 1 h before or 4 h after these drugs). An increased incidence of myopathy has been noted when lovastatin, another HMG-CoA reductase inhibitor, has been given concurrently with gemfibrozil or niacin, and thus provastatin should probably not be given concurrently with these agents.

Cautions: Contraindicated in pregnant or potentially pregnant patients.
Contraindicated in patients with active liver disease or unexplained transaminase elevations.
Use with caution in patients with history of liver disease or heavy alcohol use.

Pearls: Cost $$$ (≈$160 retail/100 tablets).
Check LFTs prior to initiating therapy, every 6 weeks for first 6 months, every 8 weeks during remainder of first year, and then at 6-month intervals.
Discontinue if persistent LFT increases >3 times normal, substantial rise in CPK, or myositis occurs.
Pregnancy category X.

PRAZOSIN (Minipress)

Dose: First dose: 1 mg PO given at night (because it can cause syncope), then begin 1 mg PO bid–tid; usual, 3–5 mg PO bid–tid; max, 20 mg PO daily.

Preparations: 1, 2, and 5 mg tablets.

Actions: α_1-Blocker that causes peripheral dilatation; used to treat hypertension.

Clearance: Metabolized via liver.
No change in dosage needed for impaired renal function.
Initial and maintenance doses should probably be reduced in liver disease.
Supplemental dose not required after HD or PD.

Side Effects: Dizziness, headache, drowsiness, fatigue, weakness, palpitations, angina, edema, orthostatic hypotension, syncope, dyspnea, nausea and vomiting, diarrhea, constipation, rash, blurred vision, reddened sclera, urinary frequency, impotence, priapism, epistaxis, nasal congestion, dry mouth, (+) ANA titer.

Pearls: Cost: generic $$, Minipress $$$ (generic ≈$0.70/d retail, Minipress ≈$1.50/d retail).
Increase dosage *slowly.*
Patients usually do *not* get reflex tachycardia.
Is especially good for lowering diastolic BP.
When adding other hypertension agents, decrease dosage to 1–2 mg tid then retitrate upward.
Pregnancy category C.

PREDNISOLONE (Delta-Cortef, Hydeltrasol, Hydeltra-T.B.A.)

Dose: Preparation dependent.
Delta-Cortef: 5–60 mg PO daily in 2–4 divided doses.
Hydeltrasol: Variable dose IM, IV, or directly into lesion or joint (large joint 10–20 mg, small joint 4–5 mg, bursae 10–15 mg, tendon sheath 2–5 mg, ganglia 5–10 mg).
Hydeltra-T.B.A.: Variable dose given q2–3wk prn IM or into lesion or joint (large joint 20–60 mg, small joint 8–10 mg, bursae 20–30 mg, ganglia 10–20 mg).

Preparations: 5 mg tablets of Delta-Cortef; 1 and 5 mg vials of Hydeltra-T.B.A. containing 20 mg/mL prednisolone tebutate; 2 and 5 mL vials of Hydeltrasol containing 20 mg/mL prednisolone sodium phosphate.

Actions: Synthetic corticosteroid with little mineralocorticoid activity; used primarily to treat inflammation and allergic conditions.

Clearance: Metabolized via liver.
No change in dosage needed for impaired renal function or liver disease.
Supplemental dose not required after HD.

Pearls: Is the liver-reduced active metabolite of prednisone.
Pregnancy category not established.

PREDNISOLONE SODIUM PHOSPHATE eye drops (Inflamase, Inflamase Forte)

Dose: Initially, instill 1 drop (written "gtt") into the conjunctival sac q1h while awake and q2h at night; when response is obtained, may reduce dosing frequency to q4h and then to tid–qid.

Preparations: : 5 and 10 mL solutions of Inflamase containing 0.125% prednisolone; 5 and 10 mL solutions of Inflamase Forte containing 1.0% prednisolone.

Actions: Topical steroid; used to treat inflammatory ophthalmic conditions.

Cautions: Contraindicated in acute herpes simplex infections.

Pearls: *Administering topical steroids to a patient who turns out to have herpes simplex is a medical disaster.* These drops should be prescribed only by experienced physicians.

PREDNISONE

Dose: Highly variable.

Preparations: 2.5, 5, 10, 20, and 50 mg tablets; 4 and 8 oz bottles containing 5 mg/5 mL (1 tsp).

Actions: Corticosteroid; used to treat inflammation or allergic reactions.

Clearance: Metabolized via liver to active metabolite prednisolone; even with significant liver disease, enough prednisolone should be produced to achieve therapeutic effects.

No change in dosage needed for impaired renal function. Supplemental dose suggested after HD.

Side Effects: Elevated serum glucose, Na^+ and water retention (which increases hypertension, edema, and CHF), heightened catabolism, worsening azotemia, psychic derangements ("steroid psychosis"). Can aggravate peptic ulcer disease, insomnia, and night terrors. Myopathy, osteoporosis, vertebral compression fractures, aseptic necrosis, hirsuitism, moon facies, and glucose intolerance can develop with chronic therapy.

Drug Interactions: Decreases hypoglycemic effect of insulin and OHAs. Increases risk of hypokalemia with K^+-depleting diuretics. Prolongs or shortens PT in patients taking warfarin. Phenobarbital and phenytoin reduce its serum level.

Pearls: Cost $ (10 mg $\approx$ $6 retail/100 tablets).

Follow serum glucose levels in patients receiving acute steroid therapy.

When switching from IV Solu-Medrol to PO prednisone during treatment of reactive airway disease, a somewhat arbitrary but commonly used initial dose is 40 mg PO qd with gradual taper. Usually taper over weeks in patients who have worse airway disease or are more steroid dependent; in patients with milder disease, taper by 5 mg daily or every several days.

Pregnancy category not established; watch newborns for signs of hypoadrenalism.

Relative activity of corticosteroids:

	Relative glucocorticoid and anti-inflammatory activity	Relative mineralocorticoid activity
cortisone	0.8	0.8
hydrocortisone	1.0	1.0
prednisone	4.0	0.8
methylprednisolone	5.0	0.5
dexamethasone	25–30	0.0

Premarin (oral conjugated estrogens)

Dose: Disease dependent.
Menopausal vasomotor symptoms: Give in 4-week cycles with 1.25 mg PO qd for 3 weeks then 1 week off.
Breast cancer palliation: 10 mg PO tid.
Osteoporosis: Give in 4-week cycles with 0.625 mg PO qd for 3 weeks then 1 week off.

Preparations: 0.3, 0.625, 0.9, 1.25, and 2.5 mg tablets.

Actions: Estrogen supplement; used to treat various hormone-responsive conditions.

Clearance: Metabolized and inactivated primarily in the liver.

Side Effects: Changes in vaginal bleeding pattern, breast tenderness and engorgement, increased risk of cardiovascular events, elevated calcium level in patients with breast cancer metastatic to bone, increased risk of gallbladder disease, GI distress, headache, depression, changes in libido.

Cautions: Use with caution in cardiovascular or circulatory disease. Contraindicated in pregnant or potentially pregnant patients.

Pearls: Cost $$ (1.25 mg ≈$45 retail/100 tablets).
Increases risk of endometrial cancer.
Pregnancy category X.

Preparation H ointment, cream, and suppositories

Dose: Manufacturer suggests applying to anal region or inserting a suppository whenever symptoms occur or 3–5 times daily, especially at night, in the morning, and after each bowel movement.

Preparations: 1 and 2 oz containers of ointment; 0.9 and 1.8 oz containers of cream; packages of 12, 24, 36, and 48 suppositories.

Actions: Preparation containing live yeast cell derivative that (manufacturer states) acts by increasing oxygen uptake of dermal tissues and facilitating collagen formation, and shark liver oil that acts as a protectant, softening and soothing tissues; used to help shrink swelling of hemorrhoidal tissue and to relieve pain and itching.

Pearls: Actual clinical efficacy is controversial.

Prilosec: see OMEPRAZOLE

Primaxin (IMIPENEM + CILASTATIN)

Dose: Delivery dependent.
  IV: 250–500 mg q6h.
  IM: 500–750 mg q12h.

Preparations: 250 and 500 mg vials for IV injection containing 250 or 500 mg of both imipenem and cilastatin; 500 and 750 mg vials for IM injection containing 500 or 750 mg of both imipenem and cilastatin.

Actions: Bactericidal antibiotic that inhibits cell wall synthesis. Good gram (+) coverage including strep, staph, and enterococci (but *not* MRSA); excellent gram (−) coverage including *P. aeruginosa* and β-lactamase–producing organisms; good anaerobic coverage including *B. fragilis*.

Clearance: Imipenem undergoes some liver metabolism but is predominantly metabolized in kidneys and renal excreted; cilastatin inhibits renal metabolism of imipenem.
  Slightly reduce dosage or increase dosing interval in impaired renal function.
  No change in dosage needed for liver disease.
  Supplemental dose suggested after HD.

Side Effects: Generally well tolerated. Rare elevation of LFTs, (+) Coombs' reaction, or yeast overgrowth. Can cause seizures when used at high doses, in renal failure, in elderly patients, or in patients with history of head trauma, seizures, or CNS pathology. Rapid infusion can cause nausea and vomiting.

Cautions: Patients allergic to β-lactams *may* have cross-sensitivity allergic reactions to imipenem.

Pearls: Cost $$$ (≈$80/d wholesale).
  Pregnancy category C.

PRIMIDONE (Mysoline)

Dose: Usual maintenance, 250 mg PO tid–qid.

Preparations: 50 and 250 mg tablets; 50 mg/mL suspension.

Actions: Anticonvulsant similar in structure to the barbiturates; used to treat tonic-clonic seizures.

Clearance: Metabolized via liver to phenobarbital; 40% excreted unchanged in urine.
Reduce dosage in impaired renal function.

Pearls: Cost $ (≈$8 retail/100 tablets).
Pregnancy category C.

Prinivil: see LISINOPRIL

Prinzide 12.5, Prinzide 25 (LISINOPRIL + HYDROCHLOROTHIAZIDE)

Dose: Usual, 1 or 2 tablets of Prinzide 12.5 or Prinzide 25 PO qd.

Preparations: Each tablet contains 20 mg lisinopril with 12.5 mg hydrochlorothiazide (Prinzide 12.5) or 25 mg hydrochlorothiazide (Prinzide 25).

Actions: Combination medication containing an ACE inhibitor (lisinopril) and a diuretic (hydrochlorothiazide); used to treat hypertension.

Side Effects: Dizziness, headache, cough, fatigue, orthostatic effects.

Cautions: Do not use as initial therapy for hypertension (must first determine whether the patient needs more than one type of antihypertensive medication and determine that the combination of ACE inhibitor and diuretic will not cause hypertension). Patients should already be taking lisinopril before this medication is begun. Contraindicated in second and third trimesters of pregnancy (because of lisinopril component).

Pearls: Cost $$$ (≈$1/d retail).
Pregnancy category D.

PROBUCOL (Lorelco)

Dose: 500 mg PO bid with meals.

Preparations: 250 and 500 mg tablets.

Actions: Cholesterol-lowering agent that reduces both LDL and HDL; used to treat hypercholesterolemia.

Side Effects: GI distress, CNS effects, dermatologic reactions, elevated LFTs, paresthesias, thrombocytopenia, eosinophilia.

Cautions: Contraindicated in patients with prolonged QT interval, recent myocardial damage, or history of ventricular arrhythmias or unexplained syncope.

Pearls: Cost $$$$ ($\approx$$2/d retail).
Obtain periodic ECGs to follow corrected QT (it can increase QT interval).
Benefits of lowering LDL levels must be weighed against possible detrimental effects of lowering HDL levels.
Pregnancy category B.

PROCAINAMIDE (Procan SR, Pronestyl)

Dose: Route and brand dependent.
IV: Loading dose, (1) 100 mg procainamide q3–5min to maximum of 1.5 g or (2) IV infusion at maximum rate of 20 mg/min (to avoid hypotension); watch for increased QRS and hypotension.
Maintenance: 2–4 mg/min.
PO (no PO load): Pronestyl, 500–1000 mg q4–6h; Procan SR: 500–1000 mg q8h.

Preparations: 250, 375, and 500 mg tablets of Pronestyl; 250, 500, 750, and 1000 mg tablets of Procan SR; 2 mL vials of procainamide containing 500 mg/mL and 10 mL vials of procainamide containing 100 mg/mL.

Actions: Type Ia antiarrhythmic; used to treat ventricular and supraventricular arrhythmias.

Clearance: Metabolized via liver; renal excreted.
Metabolite (NAPA) is active.

Moderately to markedly increase dosing interval in impaired renal function.

Sources differ on whether to reduce dosage in liver disease, so at minimum monitor serum levels carefully.

Reduce dosage in elderly patients.

Supplemental dose suggested after HD.

Side Effects: Hypotension, ventricular arrhythmias, conduction abnormalities, nausea and vomiting, SLE-like syndrome, decreased WBCs, RBCs, and platelets, tremor, insomnia.

Cautions: Contraindicated in patients with the ventricular arrhythmia torsades de pointes, SLE, or severe conduction abnormalities.

Pearls: Cost: generic $$, Procan SR $$$ (100 tablets retail: 750 mg generic SR ≈$32, 750 mg Procan SR ≈$75; IV ≈$100/d wholesale).

Give an AV blocker prior to use in atrial flutter (not fibrillation).

Some physicians follow procainamide (PA) and NAPA levels. Usual therapeutic levels differ between sources and between hospital laboratories. "Therapeutic" levels usually are given as approximately 4–8 to 4–10 mg/L.

Follow QRS (<50% increase) and corrected QT (25% increase) for best physiologic evidence of cardiotoxicity.

Pregnancy category C.

Procan SR: see PROCAINAMIDE

Procardia, Procardia XL: see NIFEDIPINE

PROCHLORPERAZINE (Compazine)

Dose: Route dependent.

PO: 5–10 mg tid–qid prn.

Long-acting PO (Spansule): Initially try 15 mg every morning or 10 mg bid; max, 20 mg bid.

IM: 5–10 mg q4–6h prn; max, 40 mg in 24 h.

PR: 25 mg bid prn.

Preparations: 5, 10, and 25 mg tablets; 10, 15, and 30 mg long-acting Compazine Spansules; 4 oz bottle of syrup containing 5 mg/mL; 2.5, 5, and 25 mg suppositories; 2 mL vials and ampules containing 5 mg/mL.

Actions: Phenothiazine that suppresses the chemoreceptor trigger zone; used to treat nausea.

Clearance: Metabolized primarily via liver.

Side Effects: Extrapyramidal symptoms, neuroleptic malignant syndrome, drowsiness, dizziness, blurred vision, dry mouth, decreased WBCs, hypotension, ECG changes, increased risk of convulsions.

Pearls: Cost $$$$ (10 mg ≈$80 retail/100 tablets; 25 mg suppositories ≈$3 each retail); generic form was recalled and none is currently available.

Pregnancy category not established, but use during pregnancy is generally not recommended.

Prokine: see GRANULOCYTE-MACROPHAGE COLONY-STIMULATING FACTOR

Proleukin: see INTERLEUKIN-2

PROMETHAZINE (Phenergan)

Dose: Use dependent.
  Nausea and vomiting: 12.5–25 mg PO, PR, IM, or IV.
  Sedation: 25–50 mg PO, PR, IM, or IV.

Preparations: 12.5, 25, and 50 mg tablets; 4 oz and 1 pint bottles of syrup containing 6.25 mg/5 mL (1 tsp); 12.5, 25, and 50 mg suppositories; 25 and 50 mg/mL injection.

Actions: Phenothiazine derivative with antihistaminic, sedative, antiemetic, and anticholinergic effects; used to treat nausea and vomiting, motion sickness, allergic reactions, and for sedation.

Clearance: Metabolized via liver.

No change in dosage needed for impaired renal function.

Dosage may need to be reduced in ESRD (because of excessive drowsiness).

Side Effects: Drowsiness, extrapyramidal reactions, anticholinergic effects.

Drug Interactions: Potentiates CNS depressant effects of other CNS depressants. Can increase extrapyramidal reactions in patients taking MAOI.

Cautions: Use with caution in patients with bone marrow depression, asthma, narrow-angle glaucoma, prostate hypertrophy, stenosing peptic ulcer, or bladder neck obstruction.

Pearls: Cost $$$ (10 mg tablets ≈$0.80 retail each; $25 mg suppository ≈$2.50 retail).

Pregnancy category C.

Pronestyl: see PROCAINAMIDE

PROPAFENONE (Rythmol)

Dose: Initial, 150 mg PO q8h for 3–4 days; usual maintenance, 150–300 mg PO tid.

Preparations: 150 and 300 mg tablets.

Actions: Type Ic antiarrhythmic structurally similar to propranolol; used to treat ventricular and supraventricular arrhythmias.

Clearance: Metabolized via liver with two patterns of metabolism: (1) $t_{1/2}$ of 2–10 h in >90% of patients and (2) 10–32 h in the remainder; metabolites may be active.

Reduce dosage in impaired renal function.

Decrease dosage to 150 mg PO q8–12h in liver disease.

Side Effects: Increased arrhythmias, dizziness, unusual taste, visual changes, nausea and vomiting, constipation, (+) ANA titer.

Drug Interactions: Raises serum levels of propranolol and metoprolol. Increases serum level of digoxin by 35%–85%. Cimetidine
raises its serum level by 20%. Quinidine causes the slow pattern
of metabolism ($t_{1/2}$ 10–32 h). Prolongs PT in patients taking warfarin.

Cautions: Use with caution in patients with CHF, conduction
abnormalities, or bronchospasm.

Pearls: Cost $$$$ ($\approx$$2.50–$4.50/d retail).
Pregnancy category C.

Propine ophthalmic solution: see DIPIVEFRIN

PROPOXYPHENE (Darvon, Darvon-N; *see also* Darvocet)

Dose: 65–100 mg PO q4h prn.

Preparations: 32 and 65 mg capsules of Darvon; 100 mg capsules of Darvon-N.

Actions: Narcotic analgesic; used to treat mild to moderate pain.

Clearance: Metabolized primarily via liver.
Reduce dosage or avoid in ESRD (active metabolites accumulate
that have dysrhythmic activity).
Decrease dosage in liver disease.
Supplemental dose not required after HD or PD.

Pearls: Cost: generic $$, Darvon $$$ (100 tablets retail: 65 mg
generic $\approx$$15, 65 mg Darvon $\approx$$40).
Subject to abuse and addiction.
Pregnancy category not established.

PROPRANOLOL (Inderal, Inderal LA)

Dose: Delivery dependent.
Regular-strength PO: Usual, 20–40 mg bid–qid.
Long-acting PO (Inderal LA): 80–160 mg qd.
IV: 1 mg q5min; some sources recommend giving first IV dose slowly.

Preparations: 10, 20, 40, 60, 80, and 90 mg tablets; 60, 80, 120, and 160 mg tablets of Inderal LA; 1 mg/mL injection.

Actions: Nonselective β-blocker; used to treat ischemic heart disease.

Clearance: Metabolized via liver.
No change in dosage needed for impaired renal function.
Reduce dosage in liver disease.
Supplemental dose not required after HD.

Side Effects: Hypotension, bradycardia, AV block, Raynaud-like symptoms, depression, fatigue, bronchospasm, impotence.

Drug Interactions: Decreases clearance of lidocaine and theophylline. Aluminum hydroxide reduces its absorption. Cimetidine raises its serum level. Phenytoin and phenobarbital increase its clearance.

Pearls: Cost $$ (Inderal ≈$0.90/d retail; Inderal LA ≈$0.70/d retail; 1 mg IV ≈$4 wholesale).
Taper dose when discontinuing (to avoid rebound reactions).
Pregnancy category C.

PROPYLTHIOURACIL (PTU)

Dose: Initial, 100–150 mg PO tid–qid. Maintenance, 50–300 mg daily, given qd–tid depending on source; one suggested maintenance regimen is 50–150 mg PO bid.

Preparations: 50 mg tablets.

Actions: Medication that inhibits synthesis of thyroid hormone and conversion of T_4 to T_3; used to treat hyperthyroidism.

Clearance: Metabolized via liver; renal excreted.
Slightly reduce dosage in impaired renal function.

Side Effects: Rash, pruritus, occasional GI discomfort, headache, arthralgia, paresthesias, rare decreased WBCs (usually during first 2 months of therapy).

Pearls: Cost $$ ($\approx$$0.50/d retail).
Pregnancy category D.

ProSom: see ESTAZOLAM

Proventil: see ALBUTEROL

Provera: see MEDROXYPROGESTERONE

Prozac: see FLUOXETINE

PSEUDOEPHEDRINE (Sudafed; see also Actifed, Robitussin-PE, Seldane-D)

Dose: 60–120 mg PO tid–qid.

Preparations: 30 and 60 mg tablets.

Actions: Oral decongestant that stimulates release of endogenous catecholamines, leading to both α and β stimulation; used to treat nasal congestion.

Cautions: Use with caution in hypertension.
Contraindicated in patients taking MAOI or tricyclics.

PSYLLIUM: see Metamucil

PTU: see PROPYLTHIOURACIL

Purinethol: see MERCAPTOPURINE

PYRAZINAMIDE (PZA)

Dose: Dosing schedules vary. Sanford's antimicrobial guide recommends a single dose of 25 mg/kg PO qd; other sources recommend 25–35 mg PO daily given in 3 or 4 divided doses. Max, 2.5–3.0 g daily.

Preparations: 500 mg tablets.

Actions: Bactericidal nicotinamide analog; used to treat mycobacterial infections (in combination with other antimycobacterial agents).

Clearance: Metabolized via liver; renal excreted.
Reduce dosage in impaired renal function.

Side Effects: Dose-related hepatotoxicity, frequent hyperuricemia, arthralgias, gastric irritation.

Cautions: Use with caution, if at all, in patients with liver disease or gout.

Pearls: Cost $$$$ (≈$3/d retail).
Check LFTs before beginning treatment.
Follow LFTs and uric acid levels.
Pregnancy category not established.

Pyridium: see PHENAZOPYRIDINE

PYRIDOXINE (VITAMIN B₆)

Dose: Use dependent.
B_6 deficiency: 10–250 mg PO qd.
Prophylactic therapy for patients taking isoniazid who are at risk for developing neuropathy: 25–50 mg PO qd.

Preparations: 10, 25, 50, 100, 200, 250, and 500 mg tablets; 100 mg/mL injection.

PZA: see PYRAZINAMIDE

QUAZEPAM (Doral)

Dose: 15 mg PO qhs; may be able to reduce dose to 7.5 mg PO qhs in some patients.

Preparations: 7.5 and 15 mg tablets.

Actions: Benzodiazepine; used as a hypnotic.

Clearance: Metabolized via liver; metabolites active.

Cautions: Contraindicated in pregnant and potentially pregnant patients.

Pearls: Cost $$ (≈$0.40/d retail).
Pregnancy category X.

Questran: see CHOLESTYRAMINE

Quinaglute: see QUINIDINE

Quinamm: see QUININE

Quinidex: see QUINIDINE

QUINAPRIL (Accupril)

Dose: Initial, 10 mg PO qd (5 mg PO qd for patients taking diuretics); maintenance, 10–80 mg PO daily in 1 or 2 divided doses.

Preparations: 10, 20, and 40 mg tablets.

Actions: ACE inhibitor; used to treat hypertension.

Clearance: De-esterified in the liver to active metabolite quinaprilat, which is eliminated primarily by renal excretion.
In impaired renal function, reduce initial dose to 2.5–5.0 mg and titrate subsequent dose to BP response.

Side Effects: Hypotension, cough, hyperkalemia, angioedema, worsening of "prerenal" renal failure, possible neutropenia (rare).

Drug Interactions: Decreases absorption of tetracycline. Can raise serum level of lithium. Diuretics can markedly increase its hypotensive effect. Concomitant use with K^+-sparing diuretics can lead to hyperkalemia.

Cautions: Contraindicated during second and third trimesters of pregnancy and in patients with history of allergic reactions to other ACE inhibitors.

Pearls: Cost $$$.
Monitor K^+ levels and kidney function during therapy.
Consider monitoring WBC count, especially in patients with preexisting renal or collagen vascular diseases (because of increased likelihood of developing ACE inhibitor related neutropenia).
Pregnancy category D.

QUINIDINE (QUINIDINE SULFATE, Quinaglute, Quinidex Extentabs)

Dose: Preparation dependent.
Quinidine sulfate: 200–400 mg q6h.
Quinaglute and Quinidex Extentabs: 324–648 mg q8–12h.
No PO loading dose.

Preparations: 100, 200, and 300 mg tablets of quinidine sulfate; 324 mg long-acting Quinaglute; Quinidex Extentabs containing 202 mg quinidine.

Actions: Type Ia antiarrhythmic; used to treat ventricular and supraventricular arrhythmias.

Clearance: Metabolized primarily via liver.
No change in dosage needed for impaired renal function.
Reduce dosage in elderly patients and in patients with liver dysfunction or decreased liver perfusion.
Supplemental dose suggested after HD or PD.

Side Effects: Nausea and vomiting, diarrhea (common and often dose limiting), liver toxicity, increased arrhythmias (especially the ventricular arrhythmia torsades de pointes), fever and viral-like syndromes, decreased WBCs, RBCs, and platelets, cinchonism.

Drug Interactions: Prolongs PT in patients taking warfarin.

Greatly increases serum level of digoxin (up to 100%). Drugs that induce hepatic enzymes decrease its serum level.

Cautions: Use with caution in AV disease.

Pearls: Cost: quinidine sulfate $$ (≈$0.50/d retail); Quinaglute: generic $$, Quinaglute $$$ (generic ≈$0.70/d retail, Quinaglute ≈$1.35/d retail).

Follow QRS and corrected QT intervals; discontinue for an increase of > 50% in the QRS interval or an increase of > 25% in the corrected QT interval.

For toxicity (i.e., greatly increased QT and QRS, torsades), may treat with lactate, bicarbonate, isoproterenol, or overdrive pacing.

Give AV blocker prior to use in atrial flutter (not fibrillation).

Pregnancy category C.

QUININE (QUININE SULFATE, Quinamm)

Dose: 260–520 mg PO qhs.

Preparations: 260 mg tablets.

Actions: Medication used to prevent and treat nocturnal leg cramps.

Clearance: Metabolized via liver; renal excreted.

Moderately reduce dosage or increase dosing interval in impaired renal function.

Supplemental dose suggested after HD but not after PD.

Side Effects: Cinchonism (tinnitus, headache, nausea and vomiting, visual changes, etc.), hemolysis, ITP.

Drug Interactions: Raises serum level of digoxin. Potentiates effects of neuromuscular blocking agents. Aluminum-containing antacids decrease its intestinal absorption. Urinary alkalizers can raise its serum level.

Cautions: Contraindicated in G6PD deficiency, optic neuritis, ITP, tinnitus, and in pregnant or potentially pregnant patients.

Pearls: Cost $ (≈$0.10/d retail).

Has cardiac effects similar to those of quinidine.

Pregnancy category X.

RAMIPRIL (Altace)

Dose: Initial, 2.5 mg PO qd (1.25 mg PO qd in patients taking diuretics, to avoid possible hypotension); maintenance, 2.5–20 mg daily given qd–bid.

Preparations: 1.25, 2.5, 5, and 10 mg capsules.

Actions: ACE inhibitor; used to treat hypertension.

Clearance: Metabolized via liver to more active metabolite ramiprilat; drug and metabolite are excreted in urine and feces.
  Reduce dosage in renal failure.

Side Effects: Rare hypotension, persistent nonproductive cough, aggravation of "prerenal" renal failure, hyperkalemia, angioedema.

Drug Interactions: Antacids reduce its absorption. Phenothiazines increase its hypotensive effects. Indomethacin decreases its hypotensive effects. Raises serum levels of digoxin and lithium. Concomitant use with allopurinol increases hypersensitivity to both agents.

Cautions: Contraindicated during second and third trimesters of pregnancy and in patients with history of angioneurotic edema.
  Use with caution, if at all, with K^+-sparing diuretics.
  Should probably not be used concurrently with K^+ supplements.

Pearls: Cost $$$ ($\approx$$1.60/d retail).
  Warn patients about possible hypotensive effects after first dose.
  Warn patients about possibility of angioedema.
  Check K^+, renal function, and WBCs during use (theoretical agranulocytosis, as with all ACE inhibitors).
  Caution patients to avoid salt substitutes (which contain K^+).
  Pregnancy category D.

RANITIDINE (Zantac)

Dose: Regimens for acute therapy include: (1) 150 mg PO bid, (2) 300 mg PO qhs, or (3) 50 mg IV q8h. Maintenance, 150 mg PO qhs.

Preparations: 150 and 300 mg tablets; 15 mg/mL syrup; 25 mg/mL injection.

Actions: H_2-blocker; used to treat peptic ulcer disease.

Clearance: Renal excreted.
   Slightly reduce dosage in impaired renal function.
   No change in dosage required for liver disease.
   Supplemental dose suggested after HD.

Side Effects: Nausea and vomiting, constipation, diarrhea, elevated LFTs, rare confusion and agitation in elderly patients, rare decreased platelets.

Drug Interactions: Magnesium- and aluminum-containing antacids, such as Maalox and Mylanta, reduce its bioavailability (give at least 2 h apart from ranitidine).

Pearls: Cost $$$–$$$$ (PO: acute therapy ≈$2.50/d retail, maintenance ≈$1.25/d retail; IV ≈$15/d wholesale).
   Gives false (+) protein results on urinalysis.
   Pregnancy category B.

Reglan: see METOCLOPRAMIDE

Relafen: see NABUMETONE

RESERPINE (Serpasil)

Dose: Initial, 0.5 mg PO qd for 1–2 weeks; if satisfactory decrease in BP is achieved, may decrease dosage to 0.1–0.25 mg PO qd.

Preparations: 0.1 and 0.25 mg tablets.

Actions: Central-acting agent that decreases HR and lowers BP by depleting catecholamine stores, which depresses sympathetic nerve function; used to treat hypertension and also for psychosis refractory to traditional antipsychotics.

Clearance: Metabolized via liver.
   No change in dosage needed for mild or moderate renal failure; avoid in ESRD (GFR <10 mL/min).
   Supplemental dose not required after HD or PD.

Side Effects: Dose-related depression, drowsiness, weakness, activation of peptic ulcer disease (increases secretion of hydrochloric acid) and ulcerative colitis, GI distress, nasal congestion, sexual dysfunction, bradycardia and arrhythmias, weight gain, edema.

Drug Interactions: Tricyclics can increase its antihypertensive effect. Can prolong effect of direct-acting amines (epinephrine, isoproterenol, phenylephrine, metaraminol). Inhibits action of indirect-acting amines (ephedrine, tyramine, amphetamines). Decreases effect of levodopa.

Cautions: Avoid concomitant use with MAOI. Contraindicated in active peptic ulcer disease, ulcerative colitis, and pheochromocytoma and in patients with depression or undergoing ECT.

Use with caution in patients with history of previous peptic ulcer disease, ulcerative colitis, or gallstones (can cause biliary colic).

Pearls: Cost $ ($\approx$$0.10/d retail).

Dose-related depression is a common and important side effect.

Some sources suggest a maximum dose of 0.5 mg PO qd, though, as noted, depression is dose related.

Is more effective when used with a diuretic or vasodilator, and several fixed-combination preparations are available.

Pregnancy category C.

Restoril: see TEMAZEPAM

Retin-A: see TRETINOIN topical cream, gel, and liquid

Retrovir: see ZIDOVUDINE

Rifadin: see RIFAMPIN

RIFAMPIN (Rifadin, Rimactane)

Dose: Disease dependent.

Tuberculosis: 600 mg PO or IV qd.

Meningococcal carrier: 600 mg PO bid for 2–4 days.

Preparations: 150 and 300 mg tablets; 600 mg vials for injection.

Actions: Semisynthetic antibiotic that binds to DNA-dependent RNA polymerase and inhibits RNA synthesis; usually used as antitubercular agent or in asymptomatic *N. meningitidis* infection.

Clearance: Metabolized to active metabolites; undergoes enterohepatic circulation.
 No change in dosage needed for impaired renal function.
 Reduce dosage in hepatic or biliary disease.
 Supplemental dose not required after HD.

Side Effects: Elevated LFTs, hepatitis and liver damage (with toxic effects potentiated by isoniazid), jaundice, decreased CBC, flu-like syndrome, hypersensitivity reactions. May make diabetes harder to control.

Drug Interactions: Can diminish effects of methadone, barbiturates, diazepam, verapamil, β-blockers, digoxin, quinidine, disopyramide, mexiletine, theophylline, anticonvulsants, OHAs, and warfarin. Is a hepatic enzyme inducer. Substantially reduces effectiveness of oral contraceptives.

Pearls: Cost $$$$ (≈$4/d retail); no generic form is available.
 Check LFTs before starting therapy and periodically during treatment.
 Warn patients that it colors urine, saliva, feces, sputum, nasal discharge, sweat, and tears orange-red, and that it can permanently stain soft contact lenses.
 Interferes with laboratory assays of vitamin B_{12} and folate.
 Pregnancy category not established.

Rimactane: *see* **RIFAMPIN**

Robinul: *see* **GLYCOPYRROLATE**

Robitussin: *see* **GUAIFENESIN** *and the following Robitussin preparations*

Robitussin A-C (GUAIFENESIN, CODEINE + ALCOHOL)

Dose: 10 mL (2 tsp) PO q4h prn.

Preparations: Each 5 mL (1 tsp) contains 100 mg guaifenesin, 10 mg codeine, and 3.5% alcohol; available in 2 oz, 4 oz, 1 pint, and 1 gallon bottles.

Actions: Combines expectorant with centrally acting narcotic that elevates the threshold for cough; used to treat persistent cough.

Cautions: Contraindicated in patients who have taken MAOI within 2 weeks.

Pearls: Warn patients of somnolent effects of codeine and that they should not drive or operate potentially dangerous machinery while taking codeine.

Robitussin-CF (GUAIFENESIN, PHENYLPROPANOLAMINE, DEXTROMETHORPHAN + ALCOHOL)

Dose: 10 mL (2 tsp) PO q4h prn.

Preparations: Each 5 mL (1 tsp) contains 100 mg guaifenesin, 12.5 mg phenylpropanolamine, 10 mg dextromethorphan, and 4.75% alcohol; available in 4, 8, and 16 oz bottles.

Actions: Combines expectorant, decongestant, and centrally acting cough suppressants; used to treat persistent cough.

Robitussin-DM (GUAIFENESIN, DEXTROMETHORPHAN + ALCOHOL)

Dose: 10 mL (2 tsp) PO q4–6h prn.

Preparations: Each 5 mL (1 tsp) contains 100 mg guaifenesin, 15 mg dextromethorphan, and 1.4% alcohol; available in 4, 8, and 12 oz bottles.

Actions: Combines expectorant and centrally acting cough suppressant; used to treat persistent cough.

Robitussin-PE (GUAIFENESIN, PSEUDOEPHEDRINE + ALCOHOL)

Dose: 10 mL (2 tsp) PO q4h prn.

Preparations: Each 5 mL (1 tsp) contains 100 mg guaifenesin, 30 mg pseudoephedrine, and 1.4% alcohol; available in 4, 8, and 16 oz bottles.

Actions: Combines expectorant and decongestant; used to treat persistent cough and nasal congestion.

Rocephin: see CEFTRIAXONE

Roferon-A: see INTERFERON

Rogaine: see MINOXIDIL

Rolaids (DIHYDROXYALUMINUM SODIUM CARBONATE)

Dose: 1 or 2 tablets hourly prn; max, 24 tablets in 24 h.

Preparations: Each tablet contains 334 mg dihydroxyaluminum sodium carbonate.

Rolaids, Calcium Rich (CALCIUM CARBONATE)

Dose: 1 or 2 tablets hourly prn; max, 14 tablets in 24 h.

Preparations: Each tablet contains 550 mg calcium carbonate.

Rolaids, Extra Strength (CALCIUM CARBONATE)

Dose: 1 or 2 tablets hourly prn; max, 8 tablets in 24 h.

Preparations: Each extra-strength tablet contains 1000 mg calcium carbonate.

Rolaids, Sodium Free (CALCIUM CARBONATE + MAGNESIUM HYDROXIDE)

Dose: 1 or 2 tablets hourly prn; max, 18 tablets in 24 h.

Preparations: Each tablet contains 317 mg calcium carbonate and 64 mg magnesium hydroxide.

Rufen: see IBUPROFEN

Rythmol: see PROPAFENONE

SALSALATE (Disalcid)

Dose: 1 g PO tid or 1.5 g PO bid; titrate according to individual response (full benefits may not be evident for 3–4 days).

Preparations: 500 and 750 mg tablets; 500 mg capsules.

Actions: Nonsteroidal anti-inflammatory agent with antipyretic and analgesic properties; used to treat inflammatory conditions.

Clearance: Undergoes esterase hydrolysis in the body and renal excretion.

Side Effects: Tinnitus, hearing impairment, nausea, rash, vertigo.

Drug Interactions: Can enhance hypoglycemic effect of OHAs. Is antagonistic to uricosuric agents.

Cautions: Use with caution in renal insufficiency or peptic ulcer disease.

Pearls: Cost $$$ ($\approx$$1.80/d retail).
Patients with ASA sensitivity rarely show cross-sensitivity.
Causes less upper GI bleeding than other NSAID.
Monitor plasma salicylate levels.
Therapeutic level is 10–30 mg/dL.
Signs and symptoms of overdose include tinnitus, vertigo, headache, confusion, drowsiness, sweating, hyperventilation, diarrhea, and vomiting.
Can lower measured T_4 level.

Acidification of urine can markedly increase its plasma level. Pregnancy category C.

Sargramostim: see GRANULOCYTE-MACROPHAGE COLONY-STIMULATING FACTOR

SCOPOLAMINE (Transderm Sc[bar]op)

Dose: Apply 1 disk to an area of intact skin behind the ear. Apply approximately 3 h prior to travel to attain adequate blood levels.

Preparations: Each disk delivers 0.5 mg of scopolamine over 3 days.

Actions: Belladonna alkaloid with antiemetic and antinauseant actions; used to treat motion sickness.

Side Effects: Dry mouth, drowsiness, confusion, disorientation.

Cautions: Use with caution in elderly patients, patients with obstruction of the pylorus or urinary bladder neck, patients with metabolic, liver, or renal failure, and patients taking drugs that have CNS effects or anticholinergic activity.

Pearls: Cost $$$ (box of 4 disks ≈$18 retail).
Pregnancy category C.

SCOPOLAMINE eye drops (Isopto Hyoscine)

Dose: Instill 1 or 2 drops (written "gtt") into the eye up to tid–qid.

Preparations: 0.25% solution.

Actions: Anticholinergic agent with cycloplegic and mydriatic activity that paralyzes sphincter and ciliary muscles; used to treat iridocyclitis.

Side Effects (systemic): Acute psychotic reactions.

Cautions: Contraindicated in glaucoma.

Pearls: Psychotic effects can be reversed by physostigmine.

To avoid systemic absorption, compress the lacrimal sac with a finger for 1 min after instilling drops.

Is often the drug of choice for iritis or significant corneal abrasions.

SECOBARBITAL (Seconal)

Dose: Delivery dependent.
PO (as hypnotic): 100 mg PO qhs.
IV: Up to 250 mg given at maximum rate of 50 mg in 15 sec.

Preparations: 100 mg Seconal Pulvules; 2 mL vials containing 50 mg/mL.

Actions: Rapidly acting barbiturate; used to induce sleep.

Clearance: Metabolized via liver; eliminated in urine and feces.

Cautions: Contraindicated in liver or kidney disease.

Pearls: Cost $ (100 mg Pulvule ≈$0.30 retail).
As noted, give IV push slowly.
Is addictive and can be habit forming.
Can cause skin ulceration if extravasated.
Pregnancy category D.

Seconal: see SECOBARBITAL

Sectral: see ACEBUTOLOL

Seldane: see TERFENADINE

Seldane-D (PSEUDOEPHEDRINE + TERFENADINE)

Dose: 1 tablet PO bid.

Preparations: Each tablet contains 120 mg pseudoephedrine and 60 mg terfenadine.

Cautions: Concurrent use of terfenadine with erythromycin or ketocunazole, and use in patients with hepatic dysfunction that interferes with terfenadine metabolism, have been associated with ventricular arrythmias and death. Therefore, terfenadine should not be prescribed under these conditions.

Actions: Combination antihistamine and decongestant; used to treat rhinorrhea.

Pearls: Cost $$$$ ($\approx$$105 retail/100 tablets).
Pregnancy category C.

Septra: see Bactrim

Serax: see OXAZEPAM

Serpasil: see RESERPINE

Silvadene: see SILVER SULFADIAZINE cream

SILVER SULFADIAZINE cream (Silvadene)

Dose: Apply thin layer to affected area qd–bid.

Preparations: 20, 50, 85, 400, and 1000 mg containers of 1% cream.

Actions: Topical sulfonamide antibiotic; used to prevent and treat burn wound infections.

Side Effects: Hypersensitivity reaction, skin discoloration, transient decrease in neutrophil levels.

Cautions: Some systemic absorption of sulfonamide can occur. Some hemolysis can occur in G6PD-deficient patients. Its use over an extensive body surface area can result in significant serum levels. Use with caution in sulfa allergy.

Pearls: Cost $$ (50 g $\approx$$9 retail).
Pregnancy category B.

SIMETHICONE (Gas-X, Mylicon, Phazyme; see also Mylanta)

Dose: 40–125 mg PO after each meal and qhs.

Preparations: 40, 80, and 125 mg tablets; 125 mg capsules.

Actions: Medication that disperses or prevents formation of mucus-surrounded gas pockets; used to treat flatulence and functional gastric bloating.

Pearls: Pregnancy category C.

Sinemet (CARBIDOPA + LEVODOPA)

Dose: Highly variable. Initial, 1 tablet PO tid of Sinemet 25/100.

Preparations: Each tablet of Sinemet 10/100, Sinemet 25/100, and Sinemet 25/250 contains 10, 25, and 25 mg carbidopa and 100, 100, and 250 mg levodopa respectively.

Actions: Antiparkinsonian medication; used to treat Parkinson's disease and Parkinson's syndrome. Levodopa crosses the blood-brain barrier and is converted to dopamine, which has antiparkinsonian effects. Carbidopa prevents non-CNS conversion of levodopa to dopamine.

Clearance: Metabolized via liver.
No change in dosage needed for impaired renal function.

Side Effects: Involuntary dyskinetic movements, CNS changes (rare), decreased WBCs, elevated LFTs, depression.

Drug Interactions: Concomitant use with sympathomimetics increases risk of arrhythmias. Concomitant use with antihypertensive agents increases risk of postural hypotension. Can cause hypertensive crisis in patients taking MAOI.

Cautions: Contraindicated in patients with narrow-angle glaucoma, history of melanoma, or taking MAOI.
May precipitate neuroleptic malignant syndrome-like complex if abruptly discontinued.
Should not be given to patients currently taking single-agent levodopa.
Use with caution in patients with history of MI, arrhythmias, or peptic ulcer disease (can cause upper GI bleeding).

Pearls: Cost $$$ (≈$1.80/d retail).
Can cause (+) Coombs' test.
Pregnancy category not established.

Slo-bid: see THEOPHYLLINE

Slo-Niacin: *see* NICOTINIC ACID
Slo-Phyllin: *see* THEOPHYLLINE

Slow-K: *see* POTASSIUM CHLORIDE

SODIUM BICARBONATE: *see* BICARBONATE

SODIUM POLYSTYRENE SULFONATE (Kayexalate)

Dose: Route dependent.
PO: 15–30 g in 50–100 mL of 20% sorbitol; may repeat q3–4h up to 4 or 5 doses in 24 h until hyperkalemia resolves.
PR: 50 g in 200 mL of 20% sorbitol; should be retained 30–60 min; may be repeated q4–6h up to 4 doses in 24 h.

Actions: Cation exchange resin that binds K^+ in exchange for other cations (usually Na^+) in the intestinal tract, removing K^+ from the body; used to treat hyperkalemia. Sorbitol serves as an osmotic laxative to decrease constipation.

Side Effects: Constipation, fecal impaction, gastric irritation. Its large Na^+ load can exacerbate CHF or peripheral edema.

Drug Interactions: May cause concretions if given with aluminum hydroxide.

Cautions: Use with caution in patients who may not tolerate the Na^+ load.

Pearls: Cost \$ ($\approx$\$100/lb wholesale).
Removes approximately 1 meq of K^+ for each gram of resin administered, and can lower serum K^+ 0.5–1.0 meq/L for each 50 g of resin administered.
Pregnancy category C.

Solu-Cortef: *see* HYDROCORTISONE

Solu-Medrol: *see* METHYLPREDNISOLONE

Soma: *see* CARISOPRODOL

SPIRONOLACTONE (Aldactone; see also Aldactazide)

Dose: 25–50 mg PO tid–qid.

Preparations: 25, 50, and 100 mg tablets.

Actions: K+-sparing diuretic that competitively inhibits aldosterone; usually used to treat ascites.

Clearance: Metabolized via liver; renal excreted.
Markedly increase dosing interval in impaired renal function; avoid in ESRD.
No change in dosage needed for liver disease.

Side Effects: Hyperkalemia, dehydration, hyponatremia, gynecomastia, hyperchloremic metabolic acidosis.

Drug Interactions: Can increase risk of digoxin toxicity.

Pearls: Cost $ (≈$0.20/d retail).
Follow serum electrolytes.
Pregnancy category not established.

Stelazine: see TRIFLUOPERAZINE

Streptase: see STREPTOKINASE

STREPTOKINASE (Kabikinase, Streptase)

Dose: Acute MI: 1,500,000 units IV over 1 hour.

Actions: Thrombolytic agent that acts with plasminogen to produce an "activator complex" which converts plasminogen to proteolytic enzyme plasmin, leading to thrombolysis; used to treat acute MI and certain other thrombotic conditions.

Clearance: Partially cleared by formation of an antigen-antibody complex; the reticuloendothelial system may also play a role in clearance.
Dosage adjustment in impaired renal function is not explicitly recommended.

Side Effects: Bleeding, reperfusion arrhythmias, hypotension (1–

10%), hypersensitivity, anaphylactoid reactions, fever (0–21%).

Cautions: Contraindicated in patients with active internal bleeding, intracranial neoplasm, or severe uncontrolled hypertension and in patients with history of CVA, CNS surgery within 2 months, or severe allergic reaction to streptokinase.

Relatively contraindicated in patients with history of cerebrovascular disease, trauma, cardiopulmonary resuscitation, serious GI bleeding, major surgery, obstetric delivery, organ biopsy, or recent puncture of noncompressible vessels and in patients with BP >180/110, high likelihood of left heart thrombus (e.g., mitral stenosis with atrial fibrillation), SBE, hemostatic defects, pregnancy, hemorrhagic retinopathy, age >75 years, septic thrombophlebitis, or occluded, infected AV cannula.

Pearls: Cost $$ (≈$200 wholesale); markedly less expensive than tPA and anistreplase (Eminase, APSAC).

Data suggest that streptokinase is as effective as tPA and anistreplase.

In certain specific cases, consider its use in treatment of pulmonary embolism, deep vein thrombosis, arterial thrombus, or embolism.

May not be effective if administered 5 days–6 months after previous use or after streptococcal infection.

Pregnancy category C.

STREPTOMYCIN

Dose: 1 g IM qd (for tuberculosis); with prolonged treatment, some sources suggest that frequency can eventually be reduced to 1 or 2 times weekly.

Preparations: 1 and 5 g vials.

Actions: Bactericidal antibiotic that inhibits protein synthesis; used to treat tuberculosis and other infections.

Clearance: Renal excreted via glomerular filtration.

Significantly reduce dosage in impaired renal function.

Side Effects: Neurotoxic reactions (including peripheral neuritis, encephalopathy, vestibular dysfunction and vertigo, and paresthesias of the face), auditory dysfunction (from damage to cranial nerve VIII), rash, fever, urticaria, angioedema, eosinophilia, neuromuscular blockade.

Cautions: Risk of severe neurotoxic reactions is sharply increased in patients with impaired renal function or prerenal azotemia.

Should not be given to pregnant or potentially pregnant patients.

Pearls: Cost $ (1 g ≈$3 wholesale).

Contains sulfite.

Sanford's antimicrobial guide suggests obtaining monthly audiograms.

Is known to cause fetal cranial nerve damage.

SUCCINYLCHOLINE

Dose: 1 mg/kg IV.

Preparations: 10 mg vials containing 20 mg/mL.

Actions: Short-acting neuromuscular blocker; used to obtain temporary neuromuscular paralysis.

Clearance: Rapidly hydrolyzed by plasma pseudocholinesterase.

SUCRALFATE (Carafate)

Dose: Use dependent.

Acute therapy: 1 g PO qid.

Maintenance, 1 g PO bid.

Preparations: 1 g tablets.

Actions: Nonsystemic medication that works locally; used to treat ulcers.

Clearance: Poorly absorbed.

Use with caution in ESRD (small amounts of aluminum are absorbed and can accumulate).

Side Effects: Constipation.

Drug Interactions: Can decrease absorption of cimetidine, ciprofloxacin, digoxin, norfloxacin, phenytoin, ranitidine, tetracycline, or theophylline when administered simultaneously.

Pearls: Cost $$$ (acute therapy ≈$2.40/d retail, maintenance ≈$1.20/d retail).
Administer at a separate time from other drugs when alterations in absorption are a concern.
Pregnancy category B.

Sudafed: see PSEUDOEPHEDRINE

SULBACTAM: see Unasyn

SULFAMETHOXAZOLE: see Bactrim

SULFASALAZINE (Azulfidine)

Dose: Usual maintenance, 2 g daily in divided doses bid–qid.

Preparations: 500 mg tablets; 1 pint oral suspension containing 250 mg/5 mL (1 tsp).

Actions: Combines 5-ASA and sulfapyridine; used to treat ulcerative colitis. Sulfasalazine's effectiveness was discovered accidentally and its mechanism of action is still not completely understood; 5-ASA is believed to be the more active and important component.

Clearance: Intestinal flora split most of the parent compound into its two components in the bowel; most of 5-ASA is eliminated in feces; most of sulfapyridine is absorbed, then metabolized in liver and excreted in urine.

Side Effects: Nausea and vomiting, anorexia, gastric distress, headache. Can color urine orange-yellow.

Cautions: Use with caution in G6PD deficiency. Contraindicated in sulfa allergy.

Pearls: Cost $$ (≈$0.50/d retail).
Warn patients of possible urine discoloration.
Pregnancy category B.

SULINDAC (Clinoril)

Dose: 150–200 mg PO bid (with food or antacids).

Preparations: 150 and 200 mg tablets.

Actions: Nonsteroidal anti-inflammatory agent with analgesic and antipyretic actions; used to treat pain and inflammation.

Clearance: Metabolized via liver.
No change in dosage needed in impaired renal function.
Reduce dosage in liver disease.

Side Effects: GI irritation, nausea, dyspepsia, upper GI bleeding, proteinuria, interstitial nephritis, nephrotic syndrome, worsening of "prerenal" renal failure, prolonged bleeding time.

Cautions: Contraindicated in patients with salicylate sensitivity or history of peptic ulcer or upper GI bleeding.
Use with caution in elderly patients.
Can cause premature closure of the ductus arteriosus when used during last trimester of pregnancy.

Pearls: Cost $$$ (≈$1.50/d retail).
Should not be used during last trimester of pregnancy.

Suprax: see CEFIXIME

Symmetrel: see AMANTADINE

Synthroid: see L-THYROXINE

T$_4$: see L-THYROXINE

Tagamet: see CIMETIDINE

Tambocor: see FLECAINIDE

TAMOXIFEN

Dose: 10–20 mg PO bid.

Preparations: 10 mg tablets.

Actions: Synthetic nonsteroidal agent with antiestrogenic properties that competes for estrogen binding sites; usually used to treat breast cancer.

Clearance: Extensively metabolized and excreted in bile and feces.
No change in dosage needed in impaired renal function.

Side Effects: Hot flashes, vaginal bleeding, menstrual irregularities, nausea and vomiting, rare myelosuppression, priapism, possible hypercalcemia.

Drug Interactions: Can increase PT in patients taking warfarin.

Cautions: Use with caution in patients with decreased WBCs or platelets.

Pearls: Cost $$$ ($\approx$$1.25/d retail).
Periodically check CBC.
Pregnancy category D.

Tapazole: see METHIMAZOLE

Tazicef: see CEFTAZIDIME

Tazidime: see CEFTAZIDIME

Tegretol: see CARBAMAZEPINE

TEMAZEPAM (Restoril)

Dose: 15–30 mg PO qhs prn.

Preparations: 15 and 30 mg capsules.

Actions: Benzodiazepine; used to treat insomnia.

Clearance: Metabolized via liver.
No change in dosage needed for impaired renal function or liver disease.

Cautions: Contraindicated in pregnant or potentially pregnant patients.

Pearls: Cost $$ (≈$0.50/d retail).
Pregnancy category X.

Tenormin: see **ATENOLOL**

Terazol: see **TERCONAZOLE vaginal cream and suppositories**

TERAZOSIN (Hytrin)

Dose: Initial, 1 mg PO qhs; gradually increase dosage. Usual, 1–5 mg PO qd. Max, 20 mg PO daily. If response is substantially diminished at 24 h, consider increasing dosage or giving bid.

Preparations: 1, 2, 5, and 10 mg tablets.

Actions: α_1-Receptor blocker that causes peripheral dilatation; used to treat hypertension.

Side Effects: Hypotension, orthostatic hypotension, dizziness, syncope, asthenia, headache, fatigue, somnolence, palpitations, nasal congestion, nausea.

Pearls: Cost $$$ (≈$1/d retail).
Caution patients about possible hypotensive effects.
Pregnancy category C.

TERBUTALINE inhaler (Brethaire)

Dose: 2 inhalations, 1 min apart, q4–6h.

Preparations: 75 mg canister, either with mouthpiece or as refill without mouthpiece, delivering at least 300 inhalations.

Actions: β-Adrenergic agonist bronchodilator; used to treat reversible obstructive airway disease.

Side Effects: (Most are related to systemic actions): arrhythmias, tachycardia, tremor, nervousness, headache, nausea, GI distress, rare but potentially fatal paradoxical bronchospasm.

Cautions: Use with caution in patients taking MAOI or tricyclics, in cardiac disease (especially CAD), hypertension, or hyperthyroidism, and in diabetes (large IV doses have been associated with worsening of diabetes and diabetic ketoacidosis).

Pearls: Cost $$$ (inhaler ≈$25 retail).
Pregnancy category B.

TERCONAZOLE vaginal cream and suppositories (Terazol 3 cream, Terazol 7 cream, Terazol 3 vaginal suppositories)

Dose: Apply full applicator intravaginally qhs for 3 days (Terazol 3) or 7 days (Terazol 7); insert 1 suppository intravaginally qhs for 3 days.

Preparations: Terazol 7 cream contains 0.4% terconazole and is available as 45 g tube with measured applicator; Terazol 3 cream contains 0.8% terconazole and is available as 20 g tube with measured applicator; each 2.5 g Terazol 3 vaginal suppository contains 80 mg terconazole.

Actions: Topical antifungal; used to treat candidiasis.

Side Effects: Headache, body pain, dysmenorrhea, abdominal or genital pain.

Pearls: Cost $$$ (Terazol 7 cream ≈$25 retail).
Pregnancy category C.

TERFENADINE (Seldane; see also Seldane-D)

Dose: 60 mg PO bid.

Preparations: 60 mg tablets.

Actions: Antihistamine; used to treat allergic conditions.

Clearance: Metabolized via liver.
No change in dosage needed for impaired renal function.

Drug Interactions: Concurrent use of terfenadine with erythromycin or ketoconazole has been associated with ventricular arrhythmias and death.

Cautions: Concurrent use of terfenadine with erythromycin or ketoconazole, and use in patients with hepatic dysfunction that interferes with terfenadine metabolism, have been associated with ventricular arrhythmias and death. Therefore, terfenadine should not be prescribed under these conditions.

Pearls: Cost $$$ (≈$1.50/d retail); similar to daily cost of astemizole (Hismanal).

Associated with less frequent drowsiness than other antihistamines.

Pregnancy category C.

Tessalon: see BENZONATATE

TETRACYCLINE

Dose: Route or disease dependent.
  PO: 250–500 mg qid, given 1 h before or 2 h after meals.
  IV: 500–1000 mg q12h.
  Chlamydia trachomatis infection: 500 mg PO qid for 7 days or longer.

Preparations: 100, 250, and 500 mg capsules; 250 and 500 mg tablets; 250 mg/5 mL (1 tsp) oral suspension; 250 and 500 mg/mL injection.

Actions: Bacteriostatic antibiotic that inhibits protein synthesis. Some gram (+) coverage including some strep and staph (but *not* enterococci); some gram (−) coverage (but frequent resistance); some anaerobic coverage (but many *B. fragilis* are resistant). Good coverage of *Mycoplasma, Rickettsia, Chlamydia,* and *Borellia burgdorferi* (Lyme disease).

Clearance: Metabolized via liver; renal excreted.
  Moderately decrease dosage in impaired renal function.
  Reduce dosage in liver dysfunction.
  Supplemental dose not required after HD or PT.

Side Effects: Yellowing of developing teeth, photosensitivity, GI distress, elevated BUN, hepatotoxicity, hypersensitivity reactions.

Can lead to azotemia, hyperphosphatemia, or acidosis in patients with impaired renal function. IV administration is associated with frequent phlebitis.

Drug Interactions: Can interfere with bactericidal actions of penicillins. Can prolong PT in patients taking warfarin. All antacids, calcium products, iron products, $NaHCO_3$, and sucralfate decrease its absorption. Concurrent use with diuretics increases BUN.

Cautions: Contraindicated in patients <8 years old and during second half of pregnancy (animal studies show embryo and fetal toxicity).

Pearls: Cost $$ ($\approx$$0.40/d retail); significantly less expensive than doxycycline and minocycline.
Doxycycline is generally better tolerated.
Should not be used during second half of pregnancy.
Caution patients to avoid intense sun exposure while taking tetryacycline.

Theo-24: see THEOPHYLLINE

Theo-Dur: see THEOPHYLLINE

Theolair: see THEOPHYLLINE

THEOPHYLLINE (Slo-bid, Slo-Phyllin, Theo-24, Theo-Dur, Theolair)

Dose: Highly variable. Initial, 300–400 mg PO or 5 mg/kg PO daily; may increase 25% q3d to maximum of 900 mg daily.

Preparations: Slo-Phyllin: 60, 125, and 250 mg tablets given bid–tid. Slo-bid: 50, 100, 200, and 300 mg capsules given bid–tid. Theo-Dur: 100, 200, 300, and 450 mg tablets given bid. Theo-24: 100, 200, 300, and 400 mg capsules given qd. Theolair: 125 and 250 mg tablets given tid–qid.

Actions: Xanthine derivative that may act by directly relaxing smooth muscles of the bronchial airways, increasing diaphragmatic contractility, and other mechanisms; used to treat reactive airway disease.

Clearance: Metabolized via liver.
  No change in dosage needed for impaired renal function.
  Reduce dosage by at least 50% in liver dysfunction.

Side Effects: Tachycardia, palpitations, arrhythmias, headache, seizures, coma, nausea and vomiting, constipation, reflux secondary to decreased lower esophageal sphincter pressure, tachypnea, rash.

Drug Interactions: Erythromycin and cimetidine prolong its $t_{1/2}$ and phenytoin shortens it. Fluoroquinolones raise its serum level.

Pearls: Cost: generic \$\$, brands \$\$\$ (generic ≈\$0.40/d retail, brands ≈\$0.75–\$1.20/d retail).
  $t_{1/2}$ is increased in COPD, cor pulmonale, CHF, liver disease, viral infections and high fevers, and in elderly patients.
  $t_{1/2}$ is decreased in smokers.
  Pregnancy category C.

Suggested Dosage Adjustments

If serum level is:

  <10 µg/mL, increase dosage 25% at 3-day intervals until "therapeutic level" or symptomatic relief is achieved.
  20–25 µg/mL, decrease dosage ≈10% and recheck after 3 days.
  25–30 µg/mL, omit next dose and decrease subsequent doses ≈25%; recheck after 3 days.
  >30 µg/mL, omit next 2 doses and decrease subsequent doses ≈50%; recheck after 3 days.

THIAMINE (VITAMIN B₁)

Dose: 100 mg PO, IM, or IV daily (usually given for 3 days to prevent Wernicke's encephalopathy).

Preparations: 10, 25, 50, 100, 250, and 500 mg tablets.

Side Effects: Burning at injection site, anaphylactic reaction.

Pearls: Cost $ (≈$5 retail/100 tablets).

For IV use, give in dilute solution or at high IV fluid rate (is often added to the liter of IV fluid the patient is already receiving).

Pregnancy category A.

THIORIDAZINE (Mellaril, Mellaril-S)

Dose: Disease dependent.

Psychotic manifestations: Usual starting dose, 50–100 mg PO tid; maintenance, 200–800 mg PO daily given in 2 or 3 divided doses.

Depression/anxiety: Usual starting dose, 25 mg PO tid; doses can vary widely, from 10 mg PO bid–qid to 50 mg PO tid–qid.

Use lower doses in elderly patients.

Preparations: 10, 15, 25, 50, 100, 150, and 200 mg tablets of Mellaril; 1 pint buttermint-flavored oral suspension of Mellaril-S containing 25 mg/5 mL (1 tsp); 1 pint buttermint-flavored oral suspension of Mellaril-S containing 100 mg/5 mL (1 tsp).

Actions: Phenothiazine that blocks postsynaptic dopamine receptors in the basal ganglia, hypothalamus, limbic system, brainstem, and medulla; used to treat psychotic disorders and depression with anxiety.

Clearance: Metabolized via liver; metabolites are active; undergoes enterohepatic recirculation and renal excretion.

Reduce dosage in impaired renal function.

Side Effects: Sedation and drowsiness, anticholinergic effects including dry mouth and blurred vision, neuroleptic malignant syndrome, tardive dyskinesia, low incidence of extrapyramidal reactions, ECG changes (corrected QT is prolonged, T wave changes), inhibition of ejaculation.

Drug Interactions: Potentiates CNS depressant effects of other C Aluminum- and magnesium-containing antacids decrease its absorption.

Cautions: Reduces the convulsive threshold.

Contraindicated in severe CNS depression or coma and in severe hypertensive or hypotensive heart disease.

Pearls: Cost: generic $$, Mellaril $$$$ (100 tablets retail: 50 mg generic ≈$10, 50 mg Mellaril ≈$60).

One source recommends against substituting generic form (based on unreliability of generic quality for this product).

Has fewer extrapyramidal side effects than some other phenothiazines.

Should be used only short term in treatment of anxiety.

Pregnancy category not established.

Thiuretic: see HYDROCHLOROTHIAZIDE

Thorazine: see CHLORPROMAZINE

L-THYROXINE (LEVOTHYROXINE, T₄, Levoxine, Synthroid)

Dose: Initial, 25–50 μg PO qd; may increase in 25 μg doses every 2–3 weeks. Usual, <200 μg qd.

Preparations: 25, 50, 75, 88, 100, 112, 125, 150, 175, 200, and 300 μg tablets.

Actions: Synthetic thyroxine supplement; used to treat hypothyroidism.

Clearance: Deiodinated to T_3, an active metabolite, in liver, kidney, and other tissues.

Side Effects: Signs and symptoms of hyperthyroidism if over-repleted.

Drug Interactions: Thyroid replacement increases sensitivity to warfarin (warfarin dose may need to be reduced). Cholestyramine binds T_4 and T_3 in the intestine (give Synthroid >5 h after cholestyramine).

Cautions: Contraindicated in uncorrected adrenocortical insufficiency.

Use with caution in patients with history of angina or MI and in elderly patients.

Pearls: Cost: generic $, Levoxine $, Synthroid $$ (generic ≈$0.06/d retail, Levoxine ≈$0.06/d wholesale, Synthroid ≈$0.20/d retail).

Symptoms of thyroid hormone toxicity include chest pain, increased HR, palpitations, excess sweating, heat intolerance, weight loss, nervousness, etc.

Adequate therapy usually results in normal levels of thyroid stimulating hormone and T_4 after 2–3 weeks of the maintenance dose.

Follow PT in patients taking warfarin.

Onset of action is 6–8 h for IV therapy and 3–5 days for PO therapy.

Will aggravate diabetes (dosage of insulin or OHA may need to be increased).

Is given in *micrograms*.

May be used during pregnancy.

Ticar: see TICARCILLIN

TICARCILLIN (Ticar; see *also* Timentin)

Dose: 3 g IV q4h; may be given IM.

Actions: Bactericidal semisynthetic penicillin that inhibits cell wall synthesis. Some gram (+) coverage including strep (some coverage for enterococci but less than with ampicillin, and *not* MRSA); some gram (−) coverage (acts synergistically with aminoglycosides against *P. aeruginosa*); good anaerobic coverage including some *B. fragilis.*

Clearance: Renal excreted.

Markedly increase dosing interval in impaired renal function.

No change in dosage needed for liver disease.

Supplemental dose suggested after HD or PD.

Side Effects: GI distress, drowsiness, rare hypersensitivity reactions, Parkinson-like syndrome, blood dyscrasias, CNS effects, elevated LFTs, jaundice.

Cautions: Contraindicated in patients with penicillin allergy.

Pearls: Cost $$$ ($\approx$$60/d wholesale).
($+$) CSF penetration with meningeal inflammation.
Carries high Na$^+$ load.
Pregnancy category not established.

Ticlid: see TICLOPIDINE

TICLOPIDINE (Ticlid)

Dose: 250 mg PO bid with food.

Preparations: 250 mg tablets.

Actions: Antiplatelet agent that causes time- and dose-dependent inhibition of both platelet aggregation and release of platelet granule constituents; used to decrease the incidence of future stroke in patients who have had transient ischemic attacks or prior thrombotic strokes and who are allergic to aspirin.

Clearance: Extensively metabolized in the liver.
Patients with moderate renal failure may have greater prolongation of bleeding time.
Should not be given in advanced liver disease (in part because of increased risk of bleeding).

Side Effects: Diarrhea, nausea, dyspepsia, rash, elevated LFTs, neutropenia, elevated total cholesterol.

Drug Interactions: Decreases elimination of theophylline. Antacids reduce its absorption. Cimetidine decreases its clearance.

Cautions: Contraindicated in neutropenia, thrombocytopenia, hemostatic disorders, active bleeding, or severe liver disease.
Use with caution in patients with lesions (such as ulcers) that are predisposed to bleeding.

Pearls: Cost $$$ ($\approx$$40/mo retail).
Giving with food increases its absorption.
Should be reserved only for patients allergic to aspirin (because of potential for drug-induced neutropenia).
Neutropenia occurs in 2.4% of patients and is usually reversible after cessation of therapy.

Monitor WBC and neutrophil count every 2 weeks for first 3 months of therapy, more frequently if absolute neutrophil counts are consistently declining or are 30% less than pretreatment values.

Platelet inhibition is irreversible for the life of the platelet.

Prolongs bleeding time; this can be normalized within 2 h by methylprednisolone 20 mg IV; platelet transfusions can also be used to reverse its effects on bleeding.

Pregnancy category B.

Tigan: see TRIMETHOBENZAMIDE

Timentin (TICARCILLIN + CLAVULANATE)

Dose: 3.1 g IV q4–6h.

Preparations: Each 3.1 g contains 3 g ticarcillin and 100 mg clavulanate.

Actions: Antibacterial agent consisting of semisynthetic penicillin and β-lactamase inhibitor (clavulanate). Good gram (+) coverage including *S. aureus, S. epidermidis,* and enterococci (but *not* MRSA); good gram (−) coverage (but *not* ticarcillin-resistant *P. aeruginosa*); good anaerobic coverage including some *B. fragilis.*

Clearance: Primarily renal excreted.

Moderately to markedly increase dosing interval in impaired renal function.

No change in dosage needed for liver disease.

Supplemental dose suggested after HD.

Side Effects: GI distress, rash and eosinophilia, blood dyscrasias, elevated LFTs.

Cautions: Contraindicated in patients with penicillin allergy.

Pearls: Cost $$$ (≈$70/d wholesale).

(+) CSF penetration with meningeal inflammation.

Causes false (+) Coombs' test and false (+) test for proteinuria.

Pregnancy category B.

TIMOLOL (Blocadren)

Dose: Disease dependent.
Hypertension: Initial, 10 mg PO bid; usual, 10–30 mg PO bid.
Post-MI prophylaxis: 10 mg PO bid.

Preparations: 5, 10, and 20 mg tablets.

Actions: Nonselective β-blocker; used to treat hypertension and as post-MI prophylaxis.

Clearance: Metabolized primarily via liver; some renal excretion.
One source states dosage adjustment is not needed in impaired renal function; another source recommends using with caution in renal disease.
Reduce dosage in liver disease.

Side Effects: Fatigue, bradycardia.

Cautions: Contraindicated in second- or third-degree heart block, bronchial asthma or COPD, severe bradycardia, and overt heart failure.

Pearls: Cost $$$ (≈$1/d retail).
Taper when discontinuing (to avoid rebound reactions).
Pregnancy category C.

TIMOLOL MALEATE eye drops (Timoptic)

Dose: 1 drop (written "gtt") qd–bid.

Preparations: 0.25 and 0.50% solution.

Actions: Nonselective β-blocker that lowers intraocular pressure by reducing formation of aqueous humor; used to treat open-angle glaucoma.

Side Effects (local): Irritation, ptosis, visual disturbances.

Side Effects (systemic): Bronchospasm, bradycardia, hypotension, fatigue, headache.

Cautions: Use with caution in patients with asthma, COPD, CHF, or cardiac conduction abnormalities.

Pearls: If pulmonary effects are going to occur, they usually begin within 30 min of administration.

Many patients with bronchospasm, cardiac disease, or both, tolerate timolol well; others have significant bronchospasm, decreased FEV_1, bradycardia, conduction abnormalities, or decompensation of CHF.

Some sources suggest that patients at risk for bronchospasm be given the first dose under surveillance and watched for about 30 min.

Pregnancy category C.

Timoptic: see TIMOLOL MALEATE eye drops

TISSUE PLASMINOGEN ACTIVATOR (ALTEPLASE, tPA, Activase)

Dose: Delivery dependent.

"Conventional schedule": 6 mg over first 2 min, then 54 mg over first hour, then 20 mg over second hour, then 20 mg over third hour (give total of 1.25 mg/kg in patients <65 kg).

"Rapid administration": 15 mg IV bolus, then 50 mg infusion over 30 min, then 35 mg over 1 h.

Regimen for Reocclusion

Protocols for reocclusion therapy vary by institution. Suggested guidelines:

Early reocclusion (<48 h): 6 mg IV bolus, then 20 mg/h IV infusion to total dose of 50 mg.

Late reocclusion (>48 h): 15 mg IV bolus, then 50 mg IV infusion over first 30 min, then 35 mg IV over 1 h for total dose of 100 mg.

Actions: Thrombolytic agent that produces clot-specific conversion of plasminogen to plasmin, causing local fibrinolysis; used to treat acute MI.

Side Effects: Bleeding (intracranial bleeding $\approx 1\%$), reperfusion arrhythmias.

Cautions: Contraindicated in patients with active internal bleeding, history of CVA, recent CNS surgery or trauma, severe uncontrolled hypertension, known bleeding diathesis, or intracranial AVM, aneurysm, or neoplasm.

Relatively contraindicated in other cerebrovascular diseases, recent GI or GU surgery, recent trauma, age >75 years, septic thrombophlebitis, occluded and infected arteriovenous cannula, acute pericarditis, SBE, hemorrhagic retinopathy, patients taking warfarin, and patients with high likelihood of left heart thrombus.

Pearls: Cost $$$$ ($2600 wholesale); streptokinase is markedly less expensive and has similar efficacy.

Begin ASA and heparin simultaneously with administration.

Pregnancy category C.

TOBRAMYCIN

Dose: Loading, 2 mg/kg; maintenance, 1–1.67 mg/kg q8h IM or IV.

Actions: Bactericidal aminoglycoside antibiotic that irreversibly inhibits protein synthesis. Excellent aerobic gram (−) coverage with variable, hospital-dependent coverage for *P. aeruginosa* (better *P. aeruginosa* coverage than with gentamicin but some nosocomial strains are resistant).

Clearance: Renal excreted.

Markedly decrease dosage or increase dosing interval in impaired renal function.

No change in dosage needed for liver disease.

Supplemental dose suggested after HD or PD.

Side Effects: Nephrotoxicity, ototoxicity, increased neuromuscular blockade, fever, rash.

Drug Interactions: Concomitant use with cephalothin, cisplatin, cyclosporine, loop diuretics, or vancomycin increases its nephrotoxicity and ototoxicity. Prolongs PT in patients taking warfarin. Penicillins can decrease its effectiveness in renal failure.

Pearls: Cost $$ (≈$25/d wholesale).

No significant CSF penetration.
Follow serum peak and trough levels.
Gentamicin is often a less expensive alternative.
Pregnancy category D.

TOCAINIDE (Tonocard)

Dose: Initial, 400 mg PO q8h; usual maintenance, 400–600 mg PO q8h or tid; max, 2400 mg PO daily.
Manufacturer notes that patients who have a therapeutic response with the tid regimen may be tried on a bid regimen if carefully monitored.

Preparations: 400 and 600 mg tablets.

Actions: Class Ib antiarrhythmic similar to lidocaine and mexiletine; used to treat ventricular arrhythmias.

Clearance: Metabolized via liver; renal excreted.
Slightly reduce dosage in impaired renal function.
Dosage may need to be lowered in patients with hepatic dysfunction (one source suggests up to 50% reduction in severe liver disease).
Supplemental dose suggested after HD.

Side Effects: Proarrhythmic effects, CNS effects (including tremor, ataxia, dizziness, vertigo, paresthesias), nausea, rare but important blood dyscrasias (substantially decreased WBCs, PMNs, platelets, and hematocrit), very rare pulmonary fibrosis.

Drug Interactions: May have additive side effects if used with lidocaine.

Pearls: Cost $$$$ (>$2.30/d retail).
Follow CBC, especially during first 12 weeks.
Pregnancy category C.

TOLAZAMIDE (Tolinase)

Dose: Initial, 100–250 mg PO qd; maintenance, 100–1000 mg PO daily. If daily dose >500 mg, should be given bid.

Preparations: 100, 250, and 500 mg tablets.

Actions: Oral hypoglycemic agent; used to treat noninsulin-dependent diabetes.

Clearance: Metabolized via liver.
No change in dosage needed in impaired renal function.

Side Effects: Hypoglycemia, elevated LFTs, skin reactions, edema, Antabuse-like reaction with alcohol.

Pearls: Cost $$ (100 tablets retail: 250 mg generic ≈$25, 250 mg Tolinase ≈$45).
Pregnancy category C.

TOLBUTAMIDE (Orinase)

Dose: 500–3000 mg daily, given in 1 or 2 divided doses.

Preparations: 250 and 500 mg tablets.

Actions: Oral hypoglycemic agent; used to treat noninsulin-dependent diabetes.

Clearance: Metabolized via liver; renal excreted.
No change in dosage needed for impaired renal function.
Supplemental dose not required after HD.

Side Effects: Hypoglycemia, skin reactions, hyponatremia.

Pearls: Cost $$ (generic ≈$0.45/d retail, Orinase ≈$0.80/d retail).
Pregnancy category C.

Tolinase: see TOLAZAMIDE

Tonocard: see TOCAINIDE

Toprol XL: [see] METOPROLOL

Toradol: see KETOROLAC

tPA: see TISSUE PLASMINOGEN ACTIVATOR

Trandate: *see* **LABETALOL**

Transderm-Nitro: *see* **NITROGLYCERIN patch**

Transderm-Scōp: *see* **SCOPOLAMINE**

TRAZODONE (Desyrel)

Dose: Initial, 150 mg PO daily in divided doses; may increase total daily dose by 50 mg every 3–4 days. Max, 400–600 mg PO daily in divided doses. Should be taken with food.

Preparations: 50, 100, 150, and 300 mg tablets.

Actions: Nontricyclic antidepressant, associated with down-regulation of β-receptors, that can inhibit serotonin uptake or potentiate behavioral changes induced by 5-hydroxytryptophan (5-HT), a serotonin precursor; used to treat depression.

Clearance: Metabolized in the liver to a 5-HT agonist metabolite.

Side Effects: Confusion, dizziness, light-headedness, sedation and drowsiness, fatigue, insomnia, incoordination, dry mouth, hypotension (especially orthostatic hypotension), priapism, increased hypotensive effects.

Drug Interactions: Can raise serum levels of digoxin or phenytoin. Dosage of concurrently administered antihypertensives may need to be reduced. Fluoxetine (Prozac) increases its serum level and toxicity if the two are administered within weeks of each other. Augments effects of warfarin.

Cautions: Can cause priapism that requires surgical intervention. Can aggravate preexisting ventricular arrhythmias.

Pearls: Cost: generic $$$, Desyrel $$$$ (generic ≈$1/d retail, Desyrel ≈$3/d retail).

Warn patients to stop the drug and seek medical advice if priapism occurs (one-third of patients who develop priapism will require surgery).

Warn patients of possible CNS effects and to avoid potentially hazardous tasks when taking the drug, at least initially.

How it reacts with MAOI is not well known.

Most patients will respond during first week of therapy and

achieve optimal response within 2 weeks; 25% of patients will require 2–4 weeks for optimal response.

Pregnancy category C.

Trental: see PENTOXIFYLLINE

TRETINOIN topical cream, gel, and liquid (Retin-A)

Dose: Initially, apply to dry cleansed skin qhs; may adjust dosage as needed.

Preparations: 0.025, 0.05, and 0.10% Retin-A cream; 0.01, 0.025, and 0.05% Retin-A gel; 0.05% Retin-A liquid also containing 55% alcohol.

Actions: Topical medication that decreases comedone formation; used to treat acne vulgaris.

Side Effects: Stinging on application, skin irritation, photosensitivity.

Pearls: Cost $$$ (tube ≈$30 retail).
Acne can appear worsened during first 4–6 weeks of therapy.
Avoid contact with mucous membranes.
Pregnancy category C.

TRIAMCINOLONE (Azmacort)

Dose: 2 inhalations tid–qid.

Preparations: 20 g package containing 60 mg triamcinolone that delivers at least 240 oral inhalations.

Actions: Anti-inflammatory aerosolized steroid; used for *chronic* treatment of bronchial asthma in patients with disease severe enough to require steroid therapy.

Side Effects: Localized *Candida* infections, hoarseness, dry or irritated throat, dry mouth. Possible systemic absorption leading to steroid-like effects and hypothalamic-pituitary-adrenal suppression.

Pearls: Cost $$$$ (inhaler ≈$34 retail).
Pregnancy category D.

TRIAMCINOLONE nasal inhaler (Nasacort)

Dose: Usual starting dose, 2 sprays in each nostril qd. If needed, may increase to a total dose of 4 sprays in each nostril daily, administered qd, bid, or qid. Some patients may be maintained on 1 spray in each nostril qd.

Preparations: 15 mg canister that delivers at least 100 sprays.

Actions: Topical steroid; used to treat allergic rhinitis.

Side Effects: Headache, sneezing, epistaxis, dry mucous membranes, nasosinus congestion, systemic absorption with resultant steroid side effects, rare candidiasis.

Pearls: Cost $$$ (inhaler ≈$38 retail).
Pregnancy category C.

TRIAMCINOLONE ACETONIDE cream, lotion, and ointment (Aristocort A, Kenalog)

Dose: Apply thin film to affected skin bid–qid.

Preparations: Aristocort A: 15 and 60 g 0.025% cream; 15, 60, and 240 g 0.1% cream; 15 g 0.5% cream; 15 and 60 g 0.1% ointment. Kenalog: 15, 80, and 240 g 0.025% cream and ointment; 15, 60, and 80 g 0.1% cream and ointment; 20 g 0.5% cream and ointment; 60 mL 0.025% lotion; 15 and 60 mL 0.1% lotion.

Actions: Topical steroid; used to treat steroid-responsive dermatologic conditions.

Side Effects: Local irritation, folliculitis, hypertrichosis, dermatitis, epidermal and dermal atrophy, adrenal axis suppression.

Cautions: Contraindicated in varicella or vaccinia.

Pearls: Cost $$ (60 g ≈$7 retail).
Occlusive dressings enhance its systemic absorption.
Pregnancy category C.

TRIAMTERENE (Dyrenium; *see also* Dyazide, Maxzide)

Dose: 100 mg PO bid.

Preparations: 50 and 100 mg capsules.

Actions: K^+-sparing diuretic; used to treat hypertension.

Clearance: Metabolized via liver; metabolites are active; some renal and biliary excretion.
Avoid in patients with GFR <10 mL/min and in liver disease.

Side Effects: Hyperkalemia, hypokalemia, nausea and vomiting, dizziness, diarrhea.

Drug Interactions: Decreases clearance of lithium. Concomitant use with ACE inhibitors, K^+ supplements, salt substitutes, or β-blockers increases risk of hyperkalemia. Raises serum level of digoxin.

Pearls: Cost $$ (≈$0.80/d retail).
Hyperkalemia is especially common in patients with GFR <30 mL/min.
Warn patients to avoid salt substitutes during use.
Interferes with catecholamine and quinidine testing.
Can aggravate megaloblastic anemia in patients with alcoholic cirrhosis.
Pregnancy category C.

TRIAZOLAM (Halcion)

Dose: 0.125–0.250 mg PO qhs.

Preparations: 0.125 and 0.250 mg tablets.

Actions: Benzodiazepine hypnotic that decreases sleep latency, increases sleep duration, and reduces the number of nocturnal awakenings; used for short-term management of insomnia.

Clearance: Metabolized via liver.
No change in dosage needed for impaired renal function or liver disease.

Side Effects: Light-headedness, dizziness, rare amnesia.

May possibly also lead to mental status changes, or changes in mood. (These possible side effects are currently very controversial.)

Drug Interactions: Potentiates CNS depressant effects of other CNS depressants. Cimetidine and erythromycin double its $t_{1/2}$ and serum level.

Cautions: Use with caution in elderly patients (consider giving half of a 0.125 mg tablet).

Contraindicated in pregnant and potentially pregnant patients.

Pearls: Cost $$ ($\approx$$0.50/d retail).

Patients can get rebound insomnia after discontinuance.

Recently banned in the United Kingdom because of concerns about side effects.

Pregnancy category X.

TRIETHANOLAMINE otic solution (Cerumenex)

Dose and Usage: (1) Tilt head at 45-degree angle; (2) fill ear canal with Cerumenex; (3) insert cotton plug; (4) allow to remain in ear 15–30 min; (4) gently flush ear with lukewarm water. Repeat this procedure if necessary.

Preparations: 6 and 12 mL bottles with dropper.

Actions: Cerumenolytic agent that emulsifies and disperses excess or impacted ear wax; used to treat excessive, symptomatic cerumen buildup in the ear.

Side Effects: Rare local dermatitis reactions.

Cautions: Contraindicated in patients with perforated tympanic membrane or otitis media.

Discontinue if sensitization or irritation occurs.

Pearls: Cost $$$ (6 mL $\approx$$17 retail, 12 mL $\approx$$26 retail).

Pregnancy category C.

TRIFLUOPERAZINE (Stelazine)

Dose: Disease dependent.

Nonpsychotic anxiety: 1–2 mg PO bid.

Acute therapy for psychotic disorder: 1–2 mg IM q4–6h prn.

Chronic therapy for psychotic disorder: Usual starting dose, 2–5 mg PO bid; some patients may require higher doses.

Preparations: 1, 2, 5, and 10 mg tablets; 2 mg/mL concentrate (for institutional use only); 10 mL vials containing 2 mg/mL for injection.

Actions: Phenothiazine derivative; used to treat psychotic disorders and nonpsychotic anxiety.

Clearance: Extensively metabolized in the liver; metabolites are active.

Side Effects: Drowsiness, dizziness, extrapyramidal reactions, fatigue and muscle weakness, dry mouth, blurred vision, neuroleptic malignant syndrome, tardive dyskinesia, ECG changes (especially Q wave and T wave changes), cholestasis.

Drug Interactions: Concomitant use with methyldopa increases BP. Phenothiazines can decrease effect of warfarin, counteract antihypertensive effects of guanethidine and related compounds, and lower the convulsive threshold. Concomitant administration of propranolol and a phenothiazine can raise serum levels of both drugs.

Cautions: Contraindicated in patients with depressed CNS state, existing blood dyscrasias or bone marrow depression, or preexisting liver disease.

Lowers the seizure threshold and can increase risk of seizures in patients taking anticonvulsants.

Can exacerbate anginal pain and orthostatic hypotension.

Pearls: Cost: generic $, Stelazine $$$$ (generic ≈$0.30/d retail, Stelazine ≈$1.50/d retail).

Should only be used short term (<12 weeks) for treatment of nonpsychotic anxiety.

Concentrate preparation contains bisulfite and should be given diluted in juice, milk, carbonated beverages, coffee, soup, or pudding.

Pregnancy category not established.

TRIHEXYPHENIDYL (Artane)

Dose: Disease and preparation dependent.

Idiopathic parkinsonism: Give 1 mg PO the first day; may then increase daily dose by 2 mg increments every 3–5 days up to total of 6–10 mg PO given in 3 divided doses (i.e., 2–3 mg PO tid). Doses should be given around mealtime (some patients tolerate it better before meals and some afterward, depending on which side effects most affect them).

Drug-induced parkinsonism: Initially give 1 mg PO; may give subsequent higher doses after several hours if needed. Total daily dose required is usually 5–15 mg PO, given in divided doses.

Concomitant use of Artane and levodopa: 3–6 mg PO daily, given in divided doses (such as 1–2 mg PO tid).

Artane Sequels: Long-acting tablets that can be given qd–bid; once the total daily dose of trihexyphenidyl is established, Artane Sequels may be substituted on a mg per mg basis to achieve total daily dose.

Preparations: 2 and 5 mg scored tablets; 16 oz elixir containing 2 mg/5 mL (1 tsp); 5 mg sustained-action Artane Sequels.

Actions: Synthetic antispasmodic; used to treat parkinsonian symptoms, particularly tremor and rigidity.

Side Effects: Common side effects that often decrease with time include dry mouth, blurred vision, dizziness, nausea, and nervousness.

Cautions: Use with caution in patients with cardiovascular, renal, or liver disease, hypertension, acute angle-closure glaucoma, benign prostatic hypertrophy, or obstructive GI disease. *Note:* These are not contraindications to use.

Pearls: Cost $$ (≈$0.50/d retail).

Patients should have gonioscopic examination and intraocular pressure monitoring at regular intervals (can raise intraocular pressure).

Do not discontinue abruptly.

Pregnancy category C.

Trilafon: *see* PERPHENAZINE

Tri-Levlen (LEVONORGESTREL + ETHINYL ESTRADIOL)

Dose: 1 tablet PO qd, preferably after dinner or qhs; with 21-day preparation, take no pills on days 22–28 then begin a new cycle.

For both 21- and 28-day preparations, take first tablet on the first day of menses. (*Note:* Other sources recommend different protocols for beginning therapy.)

Preparations: Available in 21- and 28-pill preparations. Days 1–6: 0.050 mg levonorgestrel and 0.030 mg ethinyl estradiol; days 7–11: 0.075 mg levonorgestrel and 0.040 mg ethinyl estradiol; days 12–21: 0.125 mg levonorgestrel and 0.030 mg ethinyl estradiol. Days 22–28 (with 28-day preparation): inert tablets.

Actions: Oral contraceptive with varying dose combinations; used to prevent pregnancy.

Side Effects: Serious vascular complications, menstrual changes, cervical changes, breast changes, vaginal candidiasis, hypertension, edema, weight changes, gallbladder disease, GI distress, nausea and vomiting, liver tumors, migraine headache, rash, depression, glucose intolerance, visual changes from alteration in corneal curvature, intolerance for contact lenses. Breakthrough bleeding can occur during first several months of use.

Drug Interactions: Concomitant use with antibiotics (ampicillin, chloramphenicol, isoniazid, nitrofurantoin, penicillin VK, phenytoin, rifampin, sulfonamides, tetracycline), analgesics, anxiolytics, antihistamines, migraine preparations, phenylbutazone, phenytoin, or tranquilizers can decrease its contraceptive effectiveness.

Cautions: Contraindicated in patients with thromboembolic or thrombophlebitic disorders, cardiovascular or cerebrovascular disease, vaginal bleeding of unknown cause, endometrial or other estrogen-dependent tumors, known or suspected breast cancer, jaundice, hepatic tumors, or possible pregnancy.

Cigarette smoking increases risk of serious cardiovascular complications; patients should be *strongly* advised not to smoke.

Pearls: Cost $$$ ($\approx$$20/mo retail).

Patients should undergo complete workup prior to use with special attention to history of abnormal vaginal bleeding, BP, breast examination, and pelvic examination including cervical cytology.

Pregnancy category X.

TRIMETHOBENZAMIDE (Tigan)

Dose: Delivery dependent.
PO: 250 mg tid–qid.
Suppository: 200 mg tid–qid.
IM: 200 mg (2 mL) tid–qid.

Preparations: 100 and 250 mg tablets; 200 mg suppositories; 2 mL ampules and 20 mL vials containing 100 mg/mL.

Actions: Anticholinergic agent; used to treat nausea and vomiting. Mechanism of action may be related to central effects of the chemoreceptor trigger zone.

Side Effects: Drowsiness, CNS reactions including parkinsonian symptoms.

Pearls: Cost $$$ (250 mg ≈$50 retail/100 tablets).
Pregnancy category not established.

TRIMETHOPRIM: see Bactrim

Tri-Norinyl (NORETHINDRONE + ETHINYL ESTRADIOL)

Dose: 1 pill PO qd, preferably qhs; with 21-day preparation, take no pills on days 22–28 then begin a new cycle.
Take first pill on first Sunday after onset of menses, or that Sunday if it is first day of menses.

Preparations: Available in 21- and 28-pill preparations. Days 1–12: 0.5 mg norethindrone and 0.035 mg ethinyl estradiol; days 13–21: 1.0 mg norethindrone and 0.035 mg ethinyl estradiol. Days 22–28 (with 28-pill preparations): inert ingredients.

Actions: Oral contraceptive with varying dose combinations; used to prevent pregnancy.

Side Effects: Serious vascular complications, menstrual changes, cervical changes, breast changes, vaginal candidiasis, hypertension, edema, weight changes, gallbladder disease, GI distress, nausea and vomiting, liver tumors, migraine headache, rash, depression, glucose intolerance, visual changes from alteration in corneal curvature, intolerance for contact lenses. Breakthrough bleeding can occur during first several months of use.

Drug Interactions: Concomitant use with antibiotics (ampicillin, chloramphenicol, isoniazid, nitrofurantoin, penicillin V, phenytoin, rifampin, sulfonamides, tetracycline), analgesics, anxiolytics, antihistamines, migraine preparations, phenylbutazone, phenytoin, or tranquilizers can decrease its contraceptive effectiveness.

Cautions: Contraindicated in patients with thromboembolic or thrombophlebitic disorders, cardiovascular or cerebrovascular disease, vaginal bleeding of unknown cause, endometrial or other estrogen-dependent tumors, known or suspected breast cancer, jaundice, hepatic tumors, or possible pregnancy.

Cigarette smoking increases risk of serious cardiovascular complications; patients should be *strongly* advised not to smoke.

Pearls: Cost $$$ ($\approx$$20/mo retail).

Patients should undergo complete workup prior to use with special attention to history of abnormal vaginal bleeding, BP, breast examination, and pelvic examination including cervical cytology.

Pregnancy category X.

Triphasil (LEVONORGESTREL + ETHINYL ESTRADIOL)

Dose: 1 tablet PO qd, preferably after dinner or qhs; with 21-day preparation, take no pills on days 22–28 then begin a new cycle.

For both 21- and 28-day preparations, take first tablet on the first day of menses.

If begun after discontinuance of another oral contraceptive, take first pill on first day of withdrawal bleeding.

If tablets are begun later than first day of menstruation, use an additional form of contraception for the first week.

Preparations: Available in 21- and 28-pill preparations. Days 1–6: 0.050 mg levonorgestrel and 0.030 mg ethinyl estradiol; days 7–11: 0.075 mg levonorgestrel and 0.040 mg ethinyl estradiol; days 12–21: 0.125 mg levonorgestrel and 0.030 mg ethinyl estradiol. Days 22–28 (with 28-pill preparations): inert ingredients.

Actions: Oral contraceptive with varying dose combinations; used to prevent pregnancy.

Side Effects: Serious vascular complications, menstrual changes, cervical changes, breast changes, vaginal candidiasis, hypertension, edema, weight changes, gallbladder disease, GI distress, nausea and vomiting, liver tumors, migraine headaches, rash, depression, glucose intolerance, visual changes from alteration in corneal curvature, intolerance for contact lenses. Breakthrough bleeding can occur during first several months of use.

Drug Interactions: Concomitant use with antibiotics (ampicillin, chloramphenicol, isoniazid, nitrofurantoin, penicillin VK, phenytoin, rifampin, sulfonamides, tetracycline), analgesics, anxiolytics, antihistamines, migraine preparations, phenylbutazone, phenytoin, or tranquilizers can decrease its contraceptive effectiveness.

Cautions: Contraindicated in patients with thromboembolic or thrombophlebitic disorders, cardiovascular or cerebrovascular disease, vaginal bleeding of unknown cause, endometrial or other estrogen-dependent tumors, known or suspected breast cancer, jaundice, hepatic tumors, or possible pregnancy.

Cigarette smoking increases risk of serious cardiovascular complications; patients should be *strongly* advised not to smoke.

Pearls: Cost $$$ ($\approx$$20/mo retail).

Patients should undergo complete workup prior to use with special attention to history of abnormal vaginal bleeding, BP, breast examination, and pelvic examination including cervical cytology.

Pregnancy category X.

TRIPROLIDINE: see Actifed

TROPICAMIDE (Mydriacyl)

Dose: Instill 1 drop (written "gtt") in the eye.

Preparations: 3 mL dispenser containing 1.0% solution; 15 mL dispenser containing 0.5 or 1.0% solution.

Actions: Cycloplegic agent that dilates the pupils by paralyzing ciliary and sphincter muscles; used for funduscopic examination and refraction studies.

Side Effects (local): Increased intraocular pressure, stinging, loss of accommodation and blurred vision, photophobia.

Side Effects (systemic): CNS system disturbances.

Cautions: Contraindicated in narrow-angle glaucoma. Use with caution in patients with possible increased intraocular pressure or narrow-angle glaucoma.

Pearls: Caution patients not to drive or engage in hazardous activities while pupils are dilated.

To decrease systemic absorption, compress the lacrimal sac with a finger for 1 min after instilling drops.

Pregnancy category not established.

Tums, Tums E-X antacid tablets (CALCIUM CARBONATE)

Dose: Use dependent.

Antacid: Chew 1 or 2 tablets hourly prn; max, 16 tablets in 24 h of regular Tums or Tums E-X.

Calcium supplement: 1 or 2 tablets after meals.

Preparations: Each regular-strength Tums contains 500 mg calcium carbonate; each Tums E-X contains 750 mg calcium carbonate.

Actions: Antacid and calcium supplement.

Pearls: Each regular-strength Tums provides 20%, and each Tums E-X 30%, of the adult U.S. RDA for calcium.

Tylenol: see ACETAMINOPHEN